fitness for young people

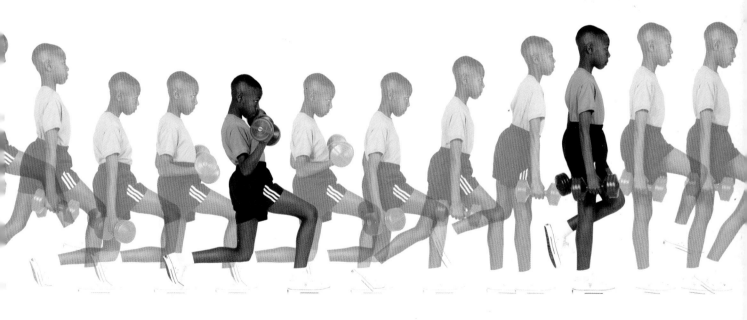

a *flow**motion*™ title

fitness for young people

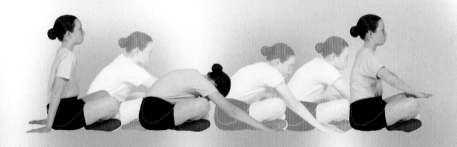

simon frost

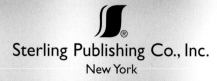

Sterling Publishing Co., Inc.
New York

Created and conceived by
Axis Publishing Limited
8c Accommodation Road
London NW11 8ED
www.axispublishing.co.uk

Creative Director: Siân Keogh
Managing Editor: Brian Burns
Design: Axis Design Editions
Editor: Antony Atha
Production Manager: Sue Bayliss
Production Controller: Juliet Brown
Photographer: Mike Good

Library of Congress Cataloging-in-Publication Data
Available

10 9 8 7 6 5 4 3 2 1

Published in 2003 by Sterling Publishing Co., Inc.
387 Park Avenue South, New York, NY 10016
Text and images © Axis Publishing Limited 2003
Distributed in Canada by Sterling Publishing
c/o Canadian Manda Group,
One Atlantic Avenue, Suite 105
Toronto, Ontario, Canada, M6K 3E7

ISBN 0–8069–9373–1

Printed by Star Standard (Pte) Limited

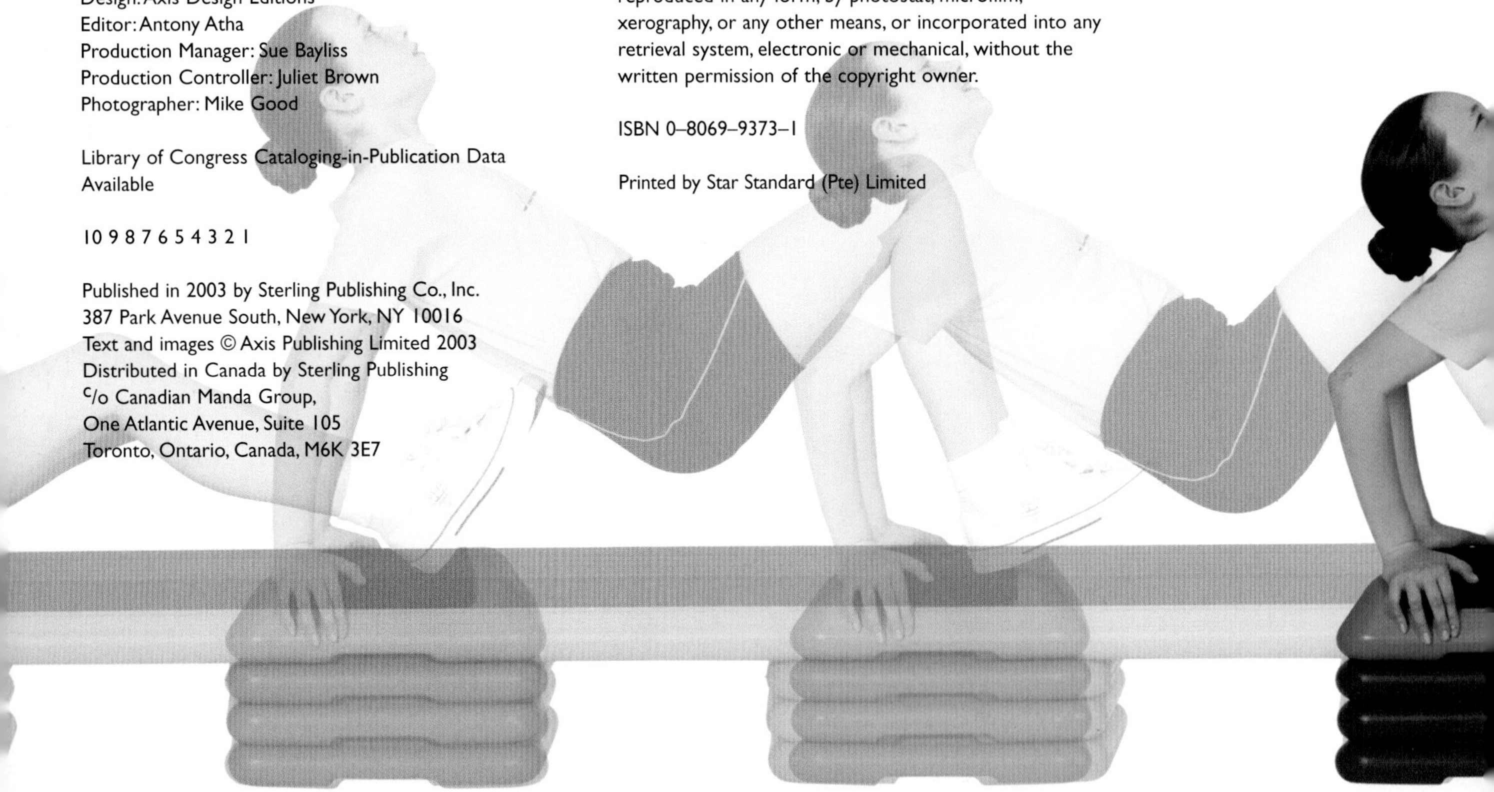

a _flow_motion™ title

fitness for young people

contents

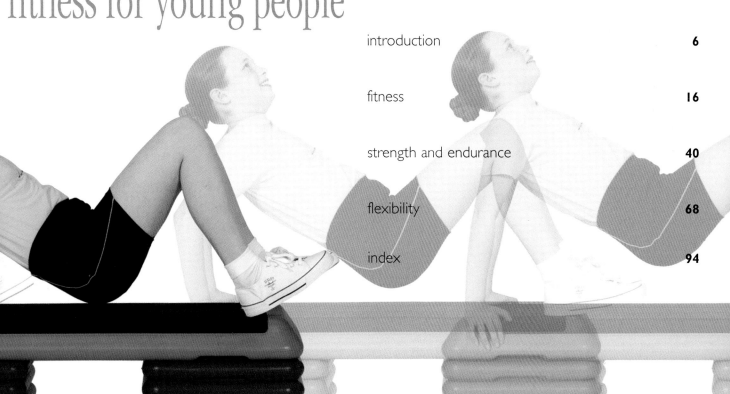

introduction

There has been a lot of research lately into children's exercise that seems to suggest that children respond to exercise in the same way that adults do. Healthy children require little encouragement to exercise—when placed in a fun environment, they are usually happy to take part in physical activities. While not everyone agrees on the sort of exercise children should be doing, how often they should be doing it, and who should be supervising, general guidelines on safety and appropriateness do exist.

The aim of this book is to let adults and children know why children between the ages of 8 and 15 should take regular exercise. It includes a wide range of safe, fun, and practical exercises that children can easily follow to achieve a new level of general fitness.

Flowmotion Fitness is divided in to three main chapters. The first, Fitness, demonstrates rhythmic exercises that increase cardiovascular fitness. The second section, Strength and Endurance, looks at exercises that can be done with simple, home-based equipment and which are designed to enhance strength and endurance. The final section, Flexibility, demonstrates how to perform specific and controlled muscle stretches to enhance overall flexibility and general body awareness.

Before and during any exercise, make sure you drink plenty of water in order to avoid becoming dehydrated.

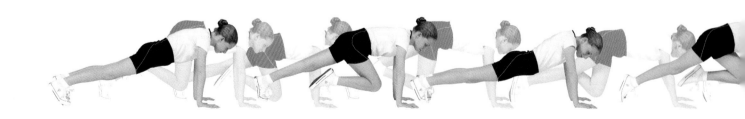

not so fit kids

Children are undeniably less fit than they used to be. Reduced physical activity affects strength, and research bears out the suggestion that the average child's strength is declining, particularly in the upper body. Lack of movement in children is also causing decreased flexibility and a significant increase in levels of obesity. And you don't have to look too far to see why.

mind over matter

Schools are reducing the time allocated for physical education to make more room for academic subjects. And more homework means there's less time for kicking a ball around the park in the evening. There is less after-school sports activity generally and since many children are travelling further to attend better schools, staying after school for team sport practice takes lower priority. When the weekend arrives, parents are often too busy to arrange or take their children to sports activities, and many children prefer to stay indoors playing video games.

safety first

Safety reasons are another factor contributing to a deterioration in levels of fitness among children. Instead of walking or even cycling to school, many children are being driven by their parents. And in many cities, parents prefer their children not to play outdoors on the streets or in local parks. Parents are also concerned that children may injure themselves if they do physical activity without supervision.

When exercising, either ask someone to watch you or use a mirror to check that your posture and form are correct.

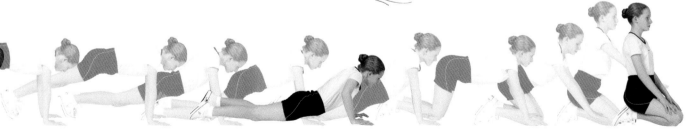

nutrition and diet

Unfortunately, an unfit, obese child is twice as likely to become an overweight or obese adult, and due to the early gains in body fat mass, there is a greater risk of suffering from medical conditions, such as coronary artery disease or Type 2 diabetes.

Inactive children tend to become inactive adults with little or no knowledge about exercise and spend a lifetime missing out on fun sports. They will most likely develop into adults who do not feel the need for, or benefits of, regular exercise and sports. That's why a massive 95 percent of adults who do lose weight are unsuccessful at keeping it off, and are far less likely to adhere to a structured health and fitness regime.

As well as psychological barriers to fitness in later life, children who don't exercise also suffer from peer pressure to be slim and good at sports. The stress this causes for girls can be overwhelming and can lead to dangerous crash dieting, comfort eating, and, in some cases, self-imposed starvation heading toward anorexia, bulimia, or both. With boys, the need to be popular with the in-crowd and the pressure to be good at sports from pushy coaches or parents can lead them to associate sport with negative emotions. And this can affect the desire to develop physical ability in the future.

so what now?

Things don't change overnight. To make a difference, adults need to encourage and motivate kids to get fit and stay fit. One way of doing this is to find out about local sports programs and facilities in your neighborhood. Take up a sport like tennis, which your child can play with you or with other children of the same ability. Ask your children what sports they enjoy or are interested in. It doesn't really matter what the sport is, as long as your kids are being active and having fun. If your child does not enjoy team sports, go to your local gym. Find a gym that runs exercise classes or junior training programs so that your child can exercise there with you or with other children.

high-fat culture

What we eat early on in life determines future dietary habits and overall health. It's very important that adults help children to improve their eating habits. Sugar, fat, and salt are the biggest problems of the modern, fast-food culture. Stop your children developing a sweet tooth by replacing sugary drinks with diluted fruit juice, and encourage them to drink water. Replace sugary snacks with fruit instead, and avoid fats, fast food, ready meals, cakes, and cookies, and commercial breakfast cereals, which are often laden with sugar. Have a look at the charts to the right, which indicate an average child's diet and the ideal diet. Compare the two and think about the changes you need to provide a good diet for your children.

With busy lifestyles, parents often resort to quick-fix meals, and school cafeterias tempt children with an array of delightful treats. This has led to a high-fat, high-calorie diet. Advertising has become more powerful, and many companies spend vast amounts of money promoting unhealthy food products, giving the impression that they are "cool." Some soft-drinks and chocolate companies even sponsor professional athletes and major sporting events.

To get the most out of training, make sure you eat a carbohydrate-based meal two to four hours beforehand.

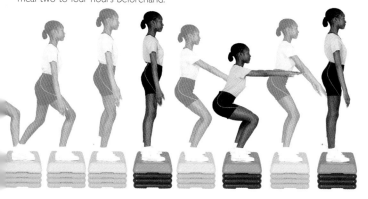

THE IDEAL DIET

The charts below show the discrepancy between the ideal diet and the average child's diet today thanks to modern eating habits.

The ideal diet

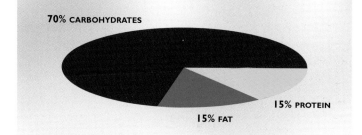

70% CARBOHYDRATES

15% PROTEIN

15% FAT

The average child's diet today

13% other 6% savory snacks 11% soft drinks 9% ice creams and sweets 14% fast food 5% meats 16% confectionery 26% cereals

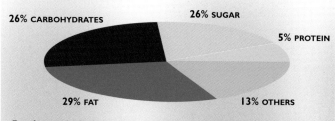

26% CARBOHYDRATES

26% SUGAR

5% PROTEIN

29% FAT

13% OTHERS

Far from ideal, the average child's diet therefore comes out as: 29% fat, 27% sugar, 26% carbohydrates, 5% protein and 13% others.

how much, how often?

To avoid injury and burnout, it's important to follow a sports schedule specially devised by a professional. My guidelines for children are as follows:

aerobic exercise

The first chapter demonstrates a range of exercises designed to increase cardiovascular fitness. Each exercise is rhythmic in nature, so they should be done at a repetitive, controlled pace to minimize the risk of injury. The step exercises require coordination and balance, which take time to master, so these should be done at walking speed to start with. The higher-impact jumping exercises may also need to be postponed until you have developed a certain level of fitness, especially if you suffer from any kind of lower-body joint problems.

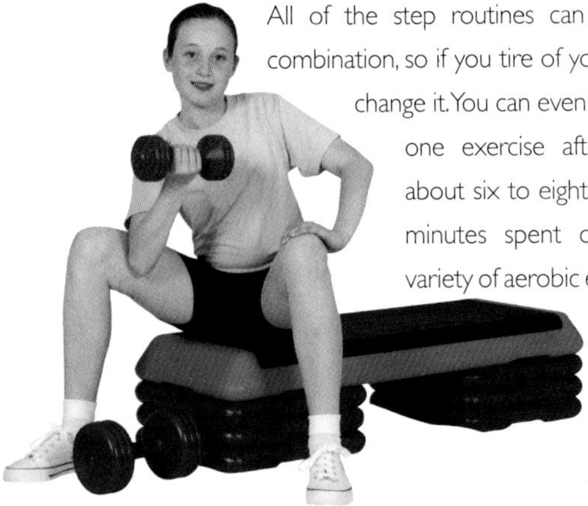

All of the step routines can be put together in any combination, so if you tire of your routine, you can always change it. You can even make up a minicircuit with one exercise after another that includes about six to eight exercises, with about two minutes spent on each. Remember, the variety of aerobic exercise is huge, and as long as you're having fun, it's not too important which exercise you choose.

LEVEL	TIME (min)
BEGINNER	5 min x 4 = 20 mins
BEGINNER	10 min x 2 = 20 mins
BEGINNER/INTERMEDIATE	15 x 2 = 30 mins
INTERMEDIATE	20–30 mins
INTERMEDIATE/IMPROVER	30–40 mins
ADVANCED	30–40 mins

*(**F**) Is for fitness *(**W**) Is for weight loss.

- Blue and Red frequency match the intensity number given to the exertion chart below.
- General fitness should not exceed 1–1½ hours per week. General weight loss should not be less than 1½ or more than 2 hours a week.
- Obese children should work up to 2–3 hours weekly, at level 2–3 intensity.

FREQUENCY (per week) (F)* OR (W)*	INTENSITY*
3 x F or 5xW	2F 2W
3 x F or 5xW	2F 3W
2–3 x F or 3–5 xW	2F 3W
3 x F or 4–5 x W	3F 2–3W
2 x F or 3–5 xW	3–4F 3–4W
2 x F or 3–5 xW	4F 2–3W

the guidelines

Children in general good health should do about 20 to 30 minutes of vigorous aerobic exercise two to three times a week. Those who are less fit may need to start with short periods of exercise and repeat them more frequently until they can comfortably do 20 minutes or more in one session. More advanced children can do 20 to 40 minutes, three to five times a week.

Start easy and progress at a steady pace. It's important that the aerobic exercise is done at a constant intensity for the total duration. Monitor the intensity using this simple talk test:

ULTRA LIGHT BREATHING NO CHANGE TO SPEECH	**not hard enough!** **increase intensity**	**1**
LIGHT BREATHING VERY LITTLE EFFECT TO SPEECH	**absolute beginner**	**2**
MEDIUM BREATHING SLIGHT PAUSES BETWEEN SPEECH	**intermediate**	**3**
HEAVY BREATHING FREQUENTLY BROKEN SPEECH	**advanced**	**4**
ULTRA-HEAVY BREATHING INCOMPREHENSIBLE SPEECH	**too hard!**	**5**

■ NEVER EXERCISE IN THE RED ZONES!

resistance training & stretching

resistance training

Using various types of equipment, children respond to resistance training much as adults do, showing significant gains in both strength and endurance. The risk associated with injury through resistance training is also low, as long as you stick to the basic do's and don'ts (see box below).

resistance training equipment

An exercise ball can be used to increase coordination, strength, and posture. The ball is very good for strengthening the torso area but it should, therefore, only be used by children who have completed at least three weeks' general conditioning.

Exercise bands are a fun way to exercise group or individual muscles and provide a challenge to all levels of fitness. Hand weights are very versatile and can be used to work any part of the body. But remember—the heavier they are, the higher the risk of injury.

DO'S AND DON'TS OF RESISTANCE TRAINING

- Seek medical clearance before allowing a child to resistance train.
- In order to minimize injury, encourage the child to express feelings of tiredness early on.
- Do not allow children to use broken or adult equipment.
- Ensure children drink plenty of water before, during, and after the exercise sessions.
- Children should be supervised while exercising.
- Make sure children are breathing properly while exercising—some have a tendency to hold their breath.
- Do not let children try to complete maximum efforts or make sudden explosive movements while exercising.
- Allow children to rest properly between sets of exercise and sessions.

RESISTANCE TRAINING CHART

LEVEL	EFFORT	NUMBER OF EXERCISES
BEGINNER	10–12 reps 1–2 sets on light resistance.	6–8 compound; multijoint exercise.
INTERMEDIATE	12–15 reps 2–3 sets on medium resistance.	10–12 compound; multijoint exercises and some possible isolated exercise.
ADVANCED	12–15 reps 2–3 sets on hard resistance.	8–10 for upper body and 6–8 for lower body, mixture of compound and isolated exercise.

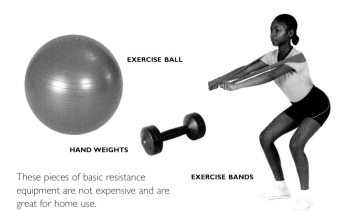

EXERCISE BALL

HAND WEIGHTS

EXERCISE BANDS

These pieces of basic resistance equipment are not expensive and are great for home use.

flexibility

Most children are not very supple, which means that they are at a higher risk of injury, postural problems, and, later in life, acute back pain. Doing simple stretches regularly really can help to prevent these problems from developing. When children stretch, it should be done gently, and each position should be held for the required length of time. The basic guideline below should help set a structured routine.

FREQUENCY	REST TIME
1–2 per week 20mins	1 min between sets and 1–2 days between sessions.
3 per week 30 mins	30 sec–1 min between sets and 1-2 days between sessions.
4 per week split routine between upper and lower body; 2 of each session; 20–30 mins per session.	30 sec–1 min between sets; 2 days on, 1 day off, then 2 days on and 2 days off (repeat).

STRETCHING CHART

LEVEL	FREQUENCY	INTENSITY	TIME	NOTES
Muscles with low flexibility	3–4 per week progressively after each session.	Low to medium pressure on each stretch.	Hold for 10–15 sec and progress to a further 3–5 per session.	Take time to stretch each muscle individually after each training session.
Muscles with medium flexibility	2–3 per week progressively after each session.	Low to medium pressure on each stretch.	Hold for 10–15secs and progress to a further 2–3 per session.	Same as above but generally stretch on non-progressive days.
Muscles with high flexibility	Generally after each session.	Low pressure on each stretch.	Hold for 10–15 secs; no progression needed.	Always stretch after training, but do not try progressive stretches.

warm up and cool down

Always build up gradually to the main exercise intensity. Spend at least five minutes before any type of exercise doing some form of light aerobic activity, and then take the time to do the following warm-up stretches. Try to stretch all the major muscles you intend to use during your workout. At the end of each workout, either do light cool-down stretches or progressive stretches, depending on your level of flexibility.

With the calf and upper back stretch, press the heel of your back foot to the ground and reach forward to increase the stretch in your upper back.

When doing the standing quadriceps, keep your knees close together and avoid touching your bottom with your foot.

This exercise stretches the chest, shoulders, and calf muscles. To increase the stretch, keep your posture upright and raise your arms higher.

The lying hamstring should be felt in the middle of the raised thigh. Keep your back flat on the floor throughout.

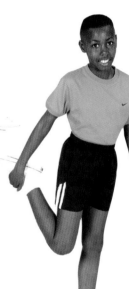

go with the flow

The special Flowmotion images used in this book have been created to ensure that you see the whole movement—not just isolated highlights. Each of the image sequences flows across the page from left to right, demonstrating how the exercise progresses and how to get into and make the most of each position safely and effectively. Each exercise is also fully explained with step-by-step captions. Below this, another layer of information in the timeline breaks the move into its various key stages, with instructions for "breathing in" and "breathing out." The symbols in the timeline also include instructions for when to pause and hold a position and when to move seamlessly from one stage to the next.

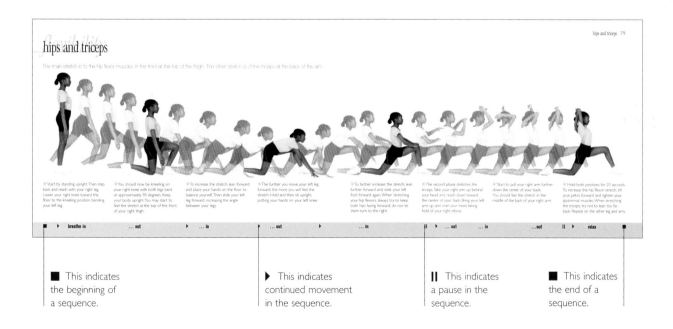

hips and triceps

The main stretch is to the hip flexor muscles in the front at the top of the thigh. The other stretch is of the triceps at the back of the arm.

● Start by standing upright. Then step back and reach with your right leg. Lower your right knee toward the floor to the kneeling position, bending your left leg.

● You should now be kneeling on your right knee with both legs bent at approximately 90 degrees. Keep your body upright. You may start to feel the stretch at the top of the front of your right thigh.

● To increase the stretch, lean forward and place your hands on the floor to balance yourself. Then slide your left leg forward, increasing the angle between your legs.

● The further you move your left leg forward, the more you will feel the stretch. Hold and then sit upright, putting your hands on your left knee.

● To further increase the stretch, lean further forward and slide your left foot forward again. When stretching your hip flexors, always try to keep both hips facing forward; do not let them turn to the right.

● The second phase stretches the triceps. Take your right arm up behind your head and reach down toward the center of your back. Bring your left arm up and over your head, taking hold of your right elbow.

● Start to pull your right arm further down the center of your back. You should feel the stretch in the middle of the back of your right arm.

● Hold both positions for 20 seconds. To increase the hip flexor stretch, tilt your pelvis forward and tighten your abdominal muscles. When stretching the triceps, try not to lean too far back. Repeat on the other leg and arm.

■ ▶ breathe in   ... out   ▶   ... in   ... out   ▶   ... in   ‖ ▶ ... out   ... in   ...out   ‖ ▶ relax   ■

■ This indicates the beginning of a sequence.

▶ This indicates continued movement in the sequence.

‖ This indicates a pause in the sequence.

■ This indicates the end of a sequence.

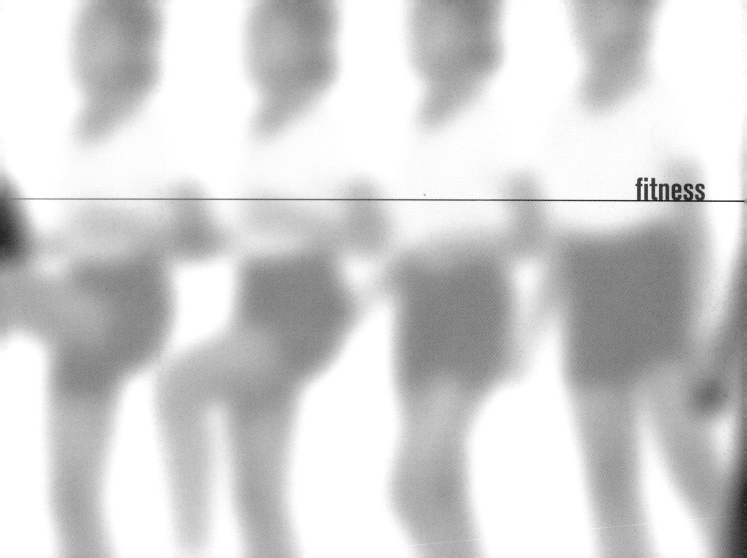

fitness

skipping

Skipping is an excellent way of increasing fitness by using all the muscles in the body, from the legs right through to the upper body, and can be done by anybody at any level. Skipping is also very good for improving coordination and is quite a low-impact exercise with minimal risk of injury.

● To start, stand in front of the rope with your feet parallel to each other, hip-width apart, your knees soft, and your hands out to the sides.

● Begin to swing the rope behind you. Looking straight ahead at the rope as it comes over your head, prepare to jump. Begin by bending from the knees, loading the body like a spring.

● Drive up through the calves and lift off the floor about 4in (10cm). Make sure that the rope is propelled by the action of your wrist in a small circular motion with minimal arm movement.

● As the rope comes into view, allow it to travel smoothly under your feet. Be careful not to over-rotate your arms, as this will create large, uneven circles rather than the desired small, rhythmic rotation

■ ▶ breathe in ▶ ... out ▶ ... in ▶

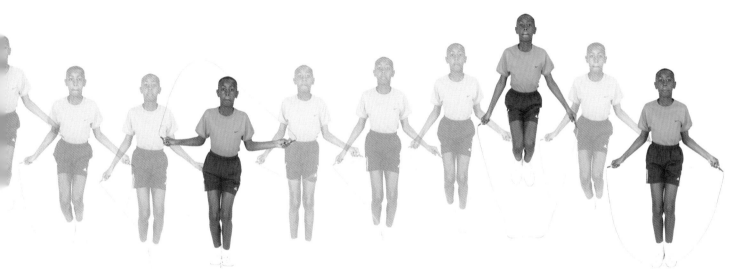

● While skipping, maintain a good upright posture. Lift from the chest, keep your head up, and avoid bending too much from the knees.

● When landing, absorb the impact first through the ankles, with soft support from the calves, landing from toe to heel. Then, absorb the impact through the knees being careful not to lock them on landing.

● Immediately, repeat the loading action of your legs to spring up into the next jump in time to the rope. Try to continue for at least five minutes. If you are skipping too fast and cannot last five minutes, then slow down.

● If it feels too easy, increase the pace in both your arms and legs or even lift your knees higher with each jump. If you are doing well, then try double skips for each jump, which is two turns of the rope for one jump.

... out   ▶   **... in**   **... out**   ▶   ■

v step box jumps

This exercise is a good way to introduce the use of a step. This very basic exercise can be combined with any number of arm movements and should be done in rhythm to music. The box step is only one exercise and can be combined with many other exercises to create a routine.

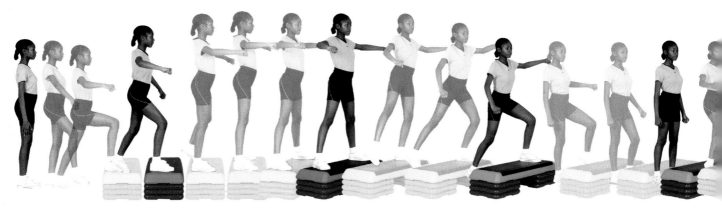

● Start in an upright posture with your feet hip-width apart. Decide on a target area and begin by raising your right foot and setting it down on the right edge of the step, in the center, with your weight evenly spread.

● Push off from your left leg, propelling yourself off the floor onto the step. Place your left foot on the left side of the step, making sure your feet are at least shoulder-width apart.

● As you raise your right foot, raise your right arm too. As your right foot hits the step, your arm should be at shoulder height. Repeat with the left foot and left arm.

● Now bring your right foot down, aiming for the same spot that you were standing on. At the same time, bring your right arm back down to your right side. Repeat with your left leg and left arm.

■   breathe in, out   ▶   … in   ▶   … out   ▶

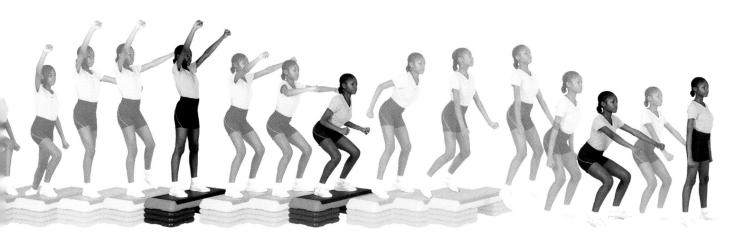

● Now repeat the step on your right foot, this time raising your right arm to punch up toward the ceiling. Drive up on your left leg while also lifting your left arm in a punch up toward the ceiling.

● With your arms in the air and your body held straight, begin to squat by bending from the thighs and pushing your bottom out behind you as if you were going to sit in a chair.

● Then bring your arms slowly down and, when your elbows are by your waist, compress your body and get ready to spring forward and up into the air. Push through your feet and jump forward off the step.

● You should land about 8–12in (20–30cm) in front of the step, your knees softly absorbing the impact and your arms out in front for balance. When landing, don't let your knees travel forward past your toes.

... in ▶ ... out ... in, out ▶ relax ■

grapevine

This all-round exercise can be combined with others to create a routine. Here it is combined with lunges, kicks, and bicep curls.

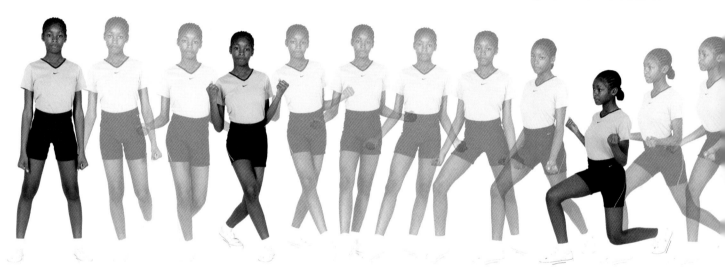

● Start with your feet a hip's width apart with your arms by your sides. Lift your left leg and step backward to the right, ending up with your left foot behind the right one and your legs crossed as shown.

● Make sure that you are well balanced and that you do not over-rotate (twist) your left knee. During the side step, begin your first bicep curl with both arms.

● As soon as you have finished the bicep curl, start to lower your arms and at the same time sweep your right foot back across your left one and out to set your position up for the lunge.

● In a lunge, your feet should be about 3ft (1m) apart, pointing in the same direction. Begin to lunge down, as shown above. Both knees should be bent at 90 degrees, and your right knee should not go beyond your toe.

 breathe in ▶ **... out** ▶ **... in** ▶ **... out**

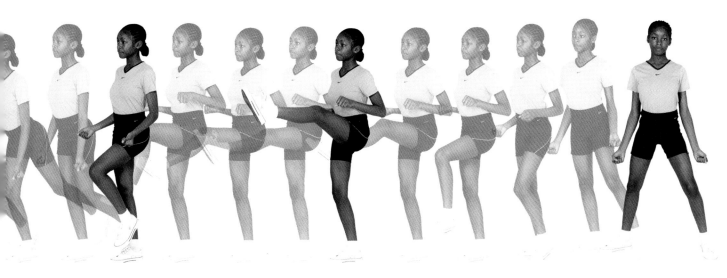

● As you lunge down, bring your arms up in a repeat bicep curl. To come out of the lunge, drive up and out, bringing your left knee toward your chest and kicking your left leg out in front. Use your arms to balance yourself.

● Kick straight out, lifting your leg as high as possible. Then start to lower your leg to the floor. Do this by bending your leg at the knee, taking your leg across and out to the side as shown in the sequence above.

● You should try to finish in the position you started from, standing facing the front with your feet apart. To make the exercise easier to start with, don't do the lunges or kicks; just do the simple side step and back to center.

● Repeat the movements in the other direction, starting with your right leg. As you get better at the exercise, build up the speed and effort.

▶   ... in   ▶   ... out   ▶   ... in   ▶   ... out, relax   ■

over box step

This simple aerobic step workout can be combined with any other step routine for a complete cardiovascular workout. If you have knee problems, do not try this exercise at speed.

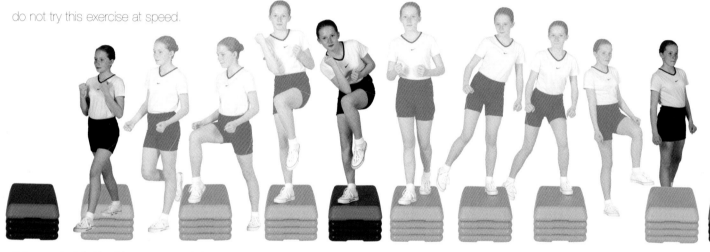

● Start on the left side of the step, with your right leg behind you. Bring your hands up and hold them tight to your chest.

● Start by stepping forward on your right leg, lowering your arms for balance. Plant your foot firmly on the step, landing toe to heel to soften the impact.

● Push off of your left leg and place your left foot on the step. Keep lifting your left leg up toward your chest while balancing on your right leg. Twist your body and touch the top of your left thigh with your right elbow.

● Try not to put your left leg down unless you are off balance. Once your elbow has touched your left thigh, bring your left leg down and place it firmly behind your right foot near the back of the step.

■   ▶   **breathe in**   **... out**   ▶   **... in**   ▶

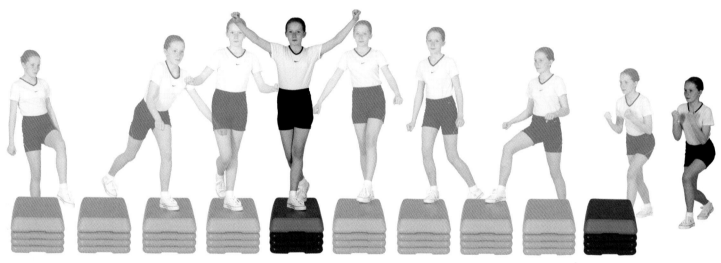

● Now, leading with your right foot, step down to the right side of the step. Follow through with your left leg, placing it back behind your right foot, and bring both arms up to your chest.

● Step back up onto the step with your left lfoot, keeping your arms down for balance. Push off your right foot to stand up on the step. As you step, lift both arms up in the air and place your right foot behind your left.

● From the start position, lower your arms for balance and, leading with your left leg, begin to step down to the left side of the step. Be careful not to twist your knees at any point.

● Once your left foot is planted, bring your right foot off the step, place it behind you, and bring both your arms up toward your chest. This whole sequence can then be repeated and mixed with other step exercises.

... out ▶ ... in ... out ▶ ... in, out, relax ■

squat lunge step

This sequence incorporates two major exercises. First, the lunge uses the muscles in the front of the thighs, hips, and calves. Then, the squat uses the muscles in the front of the thighs and the bottom.

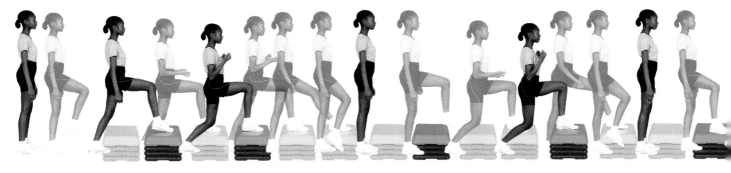

● Stand upright with your arms resting by your sides. Then place your right foot firmly upon the step. Start to raise your arms up and in toward your chest.

● As you raise your arms, slowly lower your whole body by bending at the knees. The lunge movement should be straight down, ensuring that your knee does not move forward past your toes.

● As soon as your right knee is at 90 degrees, push up and off the step with your right leg and place your right foot back on the floor. Now repeat this movement with your left leg.

● Again, once your foot is firmly upon the step, lower yourself until your left knee is at 90 degrees. Be careful not to travel forward past your toes. Then push off the step and bring your left foot back to the floor and relax.

■   ▶   breathe in, out   ▶   … in   ▶   … out   ▶

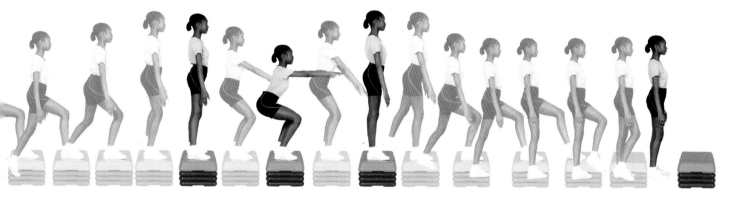

● Once again, leading with your right leg, place your foot on the step, but this time follow through with your left leg and stand upright on top of the step. Keep your feet hip-width apart.

● To begin the squat, slowly lower your body while pushing your bottom out behind, as if you were about to sit on a chair. As you squat, bring both arms up in front of you for counterbalance.

● Keep squatting and don't let your knees move forward past your toes. As soon as your knees are bent 90 degrees, drive up and out of this position until you are once more standing upright.

● Leading with your left leg, step backward off the step, taking care not to twist your ankles on landing. Bring your right foot down and place it next to your left in an upright posture.

... in   ▶   ... out   ... in   ▶   ... out, relax   ■

squat thrust push-ups

This is an advanced exercise that requires a lot of upper-body strength and whole-body endurance.

The exercise on pages 42–43, the triceps bench dips, is a good way of developing enough

strength to complete this exercise.

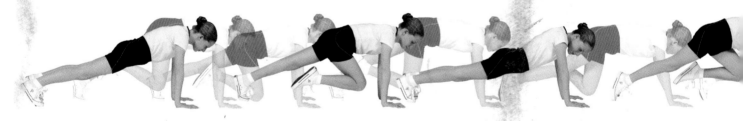

● Start in a press-up position with your hands shoulder-width apart directly under your shoulders and your feet hip-width apart. Your body should be in a straight line from head to toe.

● It is safer to do squat thrusts alternately. Start by lifting your right foot from the floor and bringing it in toward your chest, keeping your arms straight and your back flat.

● Slowly return your right foot to its starting position, so you are in press-up stance once more. While doing alternate squat thrusts, be careful not to twist your hips and put a strain on your back.

● Lift your left foot off the floor and bring your left leg in toward your chest, without it touching the floor. As soon as it touches your chest, return it to its starting position.

■   ▶   breathe in   ▶   ... out   ▶   ... in   ▶

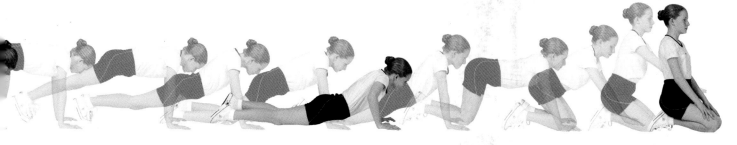

You are now ready to try the push-up. If you like, you can do more squat thrusts than prush-ups, which is less tiring for your arms. Try a ratio of three squat thrusts to one push-up.

To do a press-up, slowly bend both elbows, lowering yourself toward the floor. Try not to let your hips and stomach sink to the floor. Ideally, you should have a straight back, so keep your abs tight.

Once your elbows are at 90 degrees, begin to push back up into a straight-body position. Once you have completed the push-up, repeat the squat thrusts and so on until tired. To relax, lower your knees to the floor.

Then, using your hands, push yourself into a kneeling position with your hands upon your thighs. As this is such a tough exercise, try to build up your squat thrust to push-up ratio.

... out ▶ ... in ... out ▶ relax ■

burpee jumps

This highly aerobic exercise pushes even the fittest of children. If you are a beginner, then take your time to build up speed. To make this move less difficult, don't jump, just stand, as this will lessen the impact.

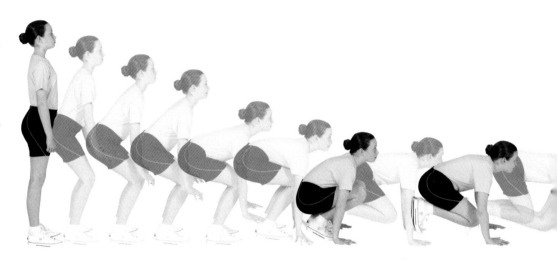

● From a firm standing position, with your arms relaxed by your sides, start to bend at both knees. Reach toward the floor with your hands but try to keep your back straight.

● Once your hands come in contact with the floor, lean forward, letting your arms take the whole of your body weight. Your hands should touch the floor a liitle in front of, and to the side of, your feet.

● With your arms fully supporting your body weight for a split second, slowly lift your feet off the floor and kick them back behind you to adopt a push-up position. This should be a smooth but fast movement.

■   ▶   **breathe in**   ▶   **... out**   ▶   **... in**   ▶

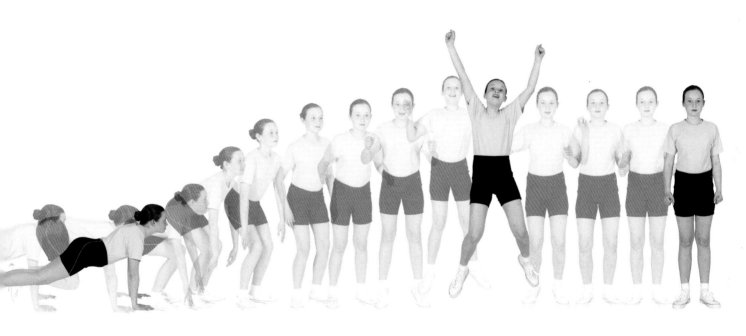

● From a prush-up position, with a spring in your legs, lift your feet off the floor and draw them back up toward your hands, bringing your knees into your chest. Again, momentarily, your arms support your whole body weight.

● From this squat position, push off your hands, bringing them up by your sides as you start to spring upward into a standing position. This exercise should be smooth and flowing, so try, if you can, not to stop at any point.

● As you drive upward, bring your arms up ready for the (optional) jump (the jump increases exercise intensity *and* the impact on your knees). Spring into the air, punching your arms out to the corners of the room.

● As you land, be careful to absorb the impact toe to heel while keeping your knees soft. Then bring your arms down by your sides and stand in an upright position to relax.

... out ▶ ... in ... out ▶ relax ■

fitness
squat star jump

This a dynamic exercise that demands lots of explosive power; it also needs a good deal of strength and is quite advanced. It is a good idea to tackle this exercise gently at first. To do this, reduce the intensity, slow it down, and don't jump too high. You can gradually build up to maximum effort and see how high you can get yourself off the ground.

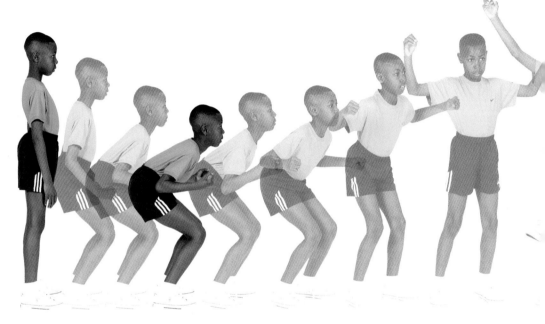

● Start by standing upright in a relaxed position with your arms by your sides. Then begin to lower your body into the squatting position. Imagine you are compressing a spring when you do this.

● Bring your arms tight in to your chest and then start to drive out and upward from the squat as quickly as possible. The faster you do this and the more power you generate, the higher the jump will be.

● As you jump, bring your arms out to your sides and lift them up toward the upper corners of the room. This helps your balance and gives your jump added impetus.

■   ▶ **breathe in**   ▶ **... out**

● As you begin your jump, spread your legs apart in the same direction as your arms. Try to move your arms and legs at the same time. Your position in the air should look like a flying star.

● It is very important that you land correctly. First, bring your arms and legs back in toward the center of your body at the same time. Try to land in the same place you took off from.

● Keep your arms bent and out to the side as shown, as this will help you to keep your balance. Flex your knees and keep your ankles loose to absorb the impact.of landing and to prevent any jarring.

● Once your feet are flat on the floor, sink down to repeat the initial squat. From here, you can either repeat the exercise or return to the relaxed starting position.

▶ … in   ▶ … out   ▶ … relax   ■

step kicks

This exercise requires flexibility, balance, and coordination. It is based on simple kickboxing type movements that in themselves are explosive and technical in execution.

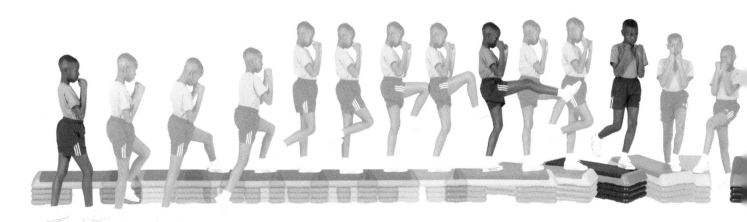

● Start in a typical boxing position with your hands up by your chin, head tucked in, body side on, and your fists closed. Your feet should be apart, right leg in front, with your weight evenly balanced between them.

● Take a step up with your left leg, placing the entire foot on the center of the step. Standing on the step, bring your right leg up, lifting your knee toward your chest. Do this quite quickly.

● When your knee is as high as it will go, begin the first kick by extending the right leg. Try to stay in the same position at all times. To stretch your leg more, try to imagine that you are kicking a target.

● Start to lower your right leg back down toward the floor but on the other side of the step from where you started. Be careful not to twist your left knee as your foot comes down toward the floor.

■ breathe in   ▶   ... in   ▶   ... out   ▶   ... in

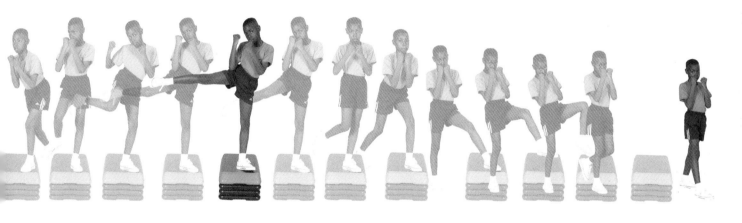

● Once your right leg has touched the floor and you are completely balanced, push up onto the step again, getting ready for the second kick. Do this as quickly as you can. Your left leg remains on the step.

● As you bring your knee up, pivot on your left foot and turn and push your right hip toward the ceiling. Be careful while doing this. Then begin the side kick with your right leg straight out as shown.

● After the full side kick, bring your right leg in and down toward your body, and then down to the floor. Pivot on your left leg and plant your right leg on the floor near the back of the step.

● Step back with your left leg and take up the starting boxing position. Be careful when doing this exercise at speed, as without rotation at the knee you could cause excessive pressure within the joint.

▶   ... in   ▶   ... out   ▶   ... in   ▶   ... out, relax   ■

touch jumps

This is another explosive exercise designed to increase the heart rate quickly. In order to do this exercise, you need to have a reasonable level of fitness. This is also a technical exercise that requires lots of coordination. When you start to practice it, make sure that you tackle it slowly at first and then aim to build up your speed gradually.

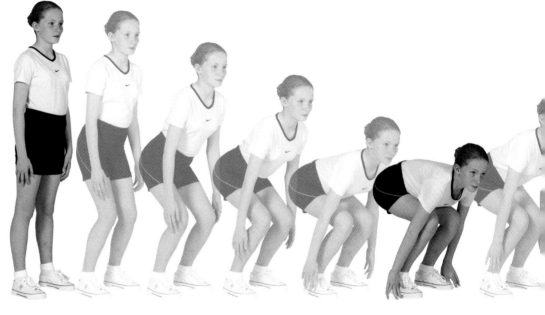

- Start standing in an upright position with your hands by your sides. Then begin to bend both knees, squatting down toward the floor. While squatting, try to keep your back straight.

- As you bend down deeper into the squat position, push your bottom back behind you but keep your head upright. Keep your back flat and lean forward to help you balance, as shown in the sequence above.

- At the bottom of the squat, at the point when your hands touch the floor, try to avoid leaning forward at the knees. They should not come forward over your toes. Push your body back and prepare to "explode."

▶ **breathe in** ▶ **... in**

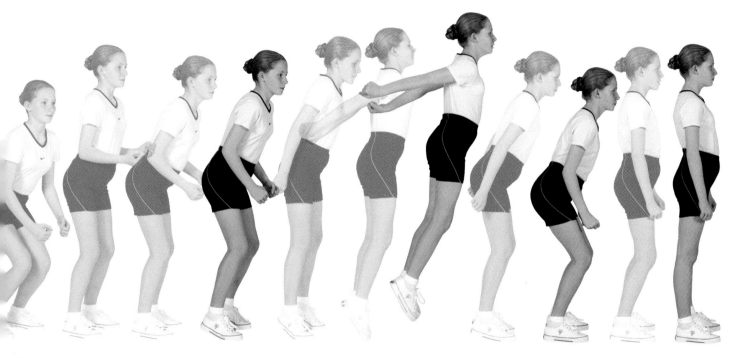

● Drive up quickly but be careful to maintain the same posture. Use your arms for balance and also to add momentum to the direction of your jump.

● You should aim to jump forward and not to jump higher than 12in (30cm). Use your arms to propel you forward and use your legs to gain height. While you are in the air, look for your landing zone.

● As you come down to the ground, begin to bend at both knees, getting ready to absorb the impact. You should do this using your muscles and not your joints.

● Land slightly on your toes at first and then begin to squat in the same way as before. Do not squat down as deeply after a jump, as this increases its intensity. If you suffer from bad knees, avoid these jumps altogether.

▶ ... out   ▶ ... out   ▶ ... in, out, relax   ■

boxercise

Shadow boxing is a fun way of fitness training. This sequence shows the four main punches.

Boxercise is very technical and requires lots of practice to achieve a good speed.

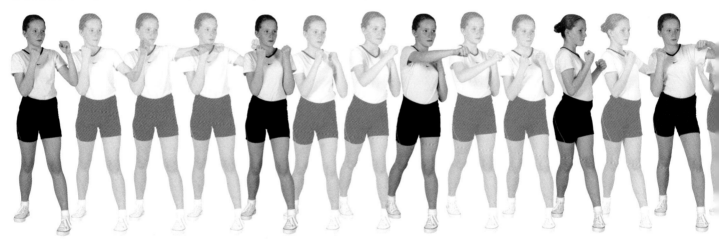

● Take up the boxing stance with your left foot in front pointing at 45 degrees to your body with your right foot 12–14in (30–40cm) behind, facing the same way. Distribute your weight evenly on the balls of both feet.

● Hold your arms on-guard up by your cheek bones, head down, fists closed. Then start your first "jab." A jab is a leading hand movement, in this case, the left. Punch out straight with your left hand and return it quickly.

● Keeping the same stance, next try a "cross." Here, your fist travels across your body and is twisted at 90 degrees as shown. Try to hit the same imaginary spot as you did with the jab, extending and returning your right arm.

● Next try a "hook" with your left hand. First twist your body away from the target, then back toward it, bringing your left arm up and around, bent at the elbow (to form the hook) and parallel to the floor.

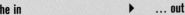 **breathe in**   ▶ **... out**   ▶ **... in**   ▶ **... out**

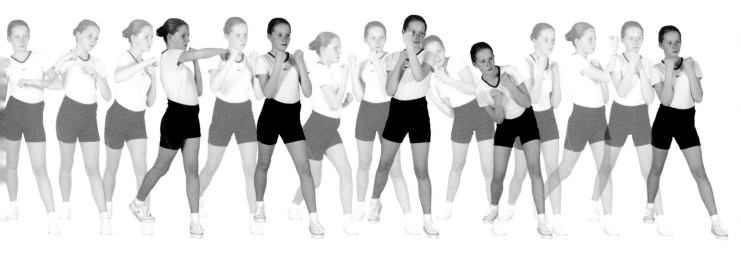

● Once the target has been hit, bring your arm down quickly to the on-guard position. Repeat the hook with your right hand in the same way. This should seem a much harder punch.

● Now try a left-hand upper cut. First, bend from the legs to sink down below the target and twist away from it, lowering your guard slightly. As you turn back toward the target, drive up with your legs and punch upward.

● When you have completed the punch, return to the on-guard position quickly. Repeat the upper cut this time using your right hand. Once you have hit the target, return to the original stance.

● When you have mastered the punches, try putting them together in different combinations, for example, jab, cross; jab, cross, left hook; or right upper cut, left hook, cross. Make up your own combinations.

▶ **... in**   ▶ **... out**   ▶ **... in**   ▶ **... out, relax**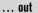

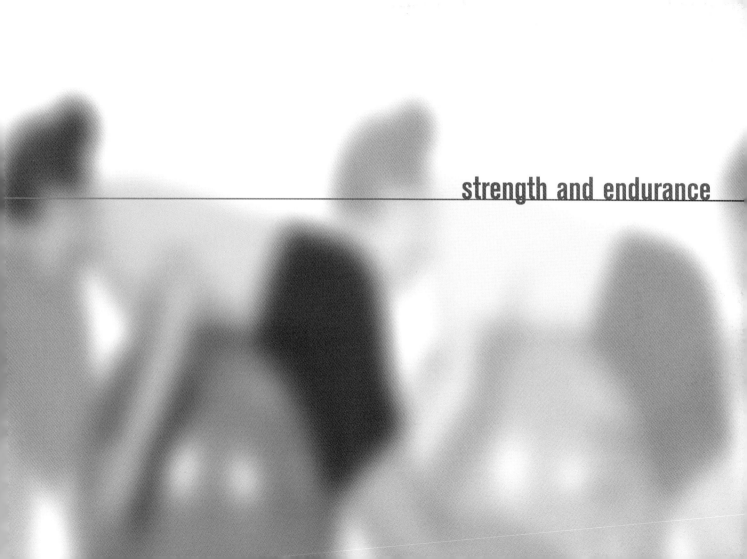

strength and endurance

tricep bench dips

This is a simple but effective exercise to develop strength and endurance in the tricep muscle of the upper back of arm. It can be done anywhere and does not require any special equipment.

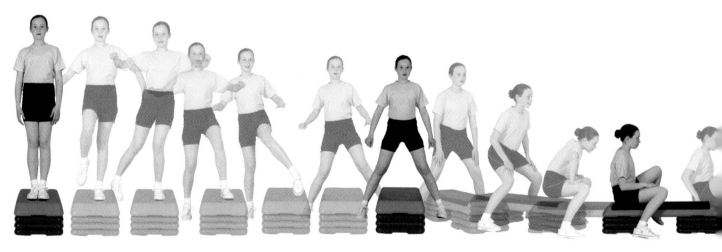

● This sequence shows how you can incorporate a number of different exercises together. Start standing on a step or box and step down with your right leg first; use your arms for balance.

● Once your right foot is on the floor and you are properly balanced, step across to the other side of the step with your left leg. You should now be in a v-step position with the step between your legs.

● Now start to squat down slowly, move your body weight back, and, at the same time, lean forward from your waist to help you keep your balance. You should be aiming to sit near the end of the step.

● Once you are seated, lift your left leg and place it on the step. Repeat this with your right leg: make sure the heels of both feet are resting on the step and that they are an even distance apart.

■ ▶ **breathe in** ▶ **... out** ▶ **... in** ▶ **... out**

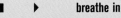
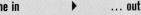
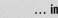

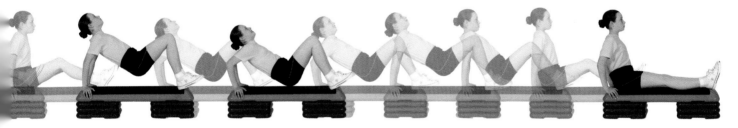

● Place your hands on either side of the step near the back. Slide your bottom forward toward your feet until the center of your body is in the middle of the step.

● Once the angle of your arms at the elbow has reached about 90 degrees, start to lift yourself up by straightening both arms but do not lock your elbows at the top of this movement—keep them soft and supple.

● Straighten your arms to lift your bottom off the step. You should aim to keep your body rigid, bending both elbows to lower and raise yourself on the step.

● Repeat this exercise as many times as you wish or until tired. Then rest by lowering your bottom onto the step. Slowly slide yourself back to the sitting position and relax.

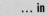 ... in    ... in   ▶ ... out    ... out, relax ■

shoulder raise and squats

There are two movements involved: one is an upper body shoulder exercise; the second is a major lower body general exercise.

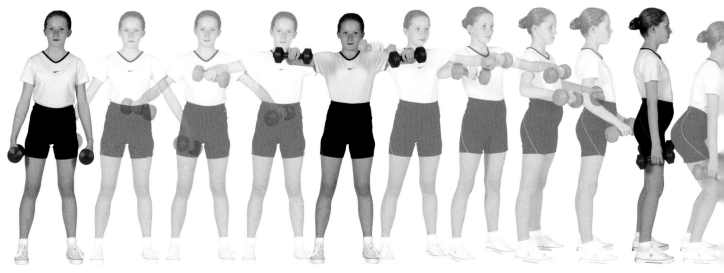

● Stand upright with your hands by your sides and your feet a hip's width apart, holding suitable weights. Raise both arms slowly out to each side at the same time. As you do so, bend your elbows.

● Aim to make a right angle with your arms at the elbow. If your arms are extended out further, this will make the exercise harder. Be careful not to put any strain on your back.

● Raise your arms until they are at shoulder height. Then pause for a second before lowering your arms down to your sides. This should be done in a slow, controlled movement. Keep your elbows soft throughout.

● Repeat as often as required or rest with your arms by your sides. To begin the squat, push your lower body backward and at the same time lean forward with your upper body to compensate for the change in balance.

■ ▶ **breathe in**   ▶ **... out**   ❚❚ **... in**

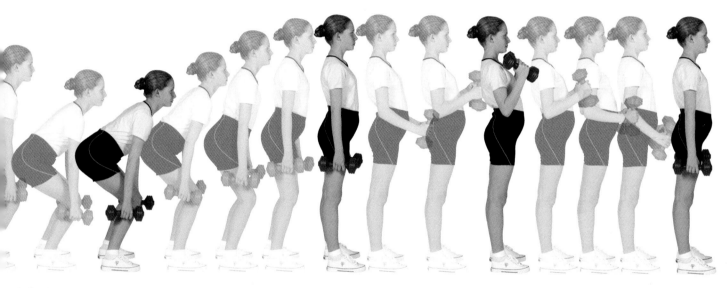

● Continue squatting, keeping your head and shoulders upright; aim to keep your back straight. Do not squat lower than 90 degrees at the knees.

● Now begin to drive up out of the squat. Keep in mind all the key elements—back, shoulders, and head. Once you are standing straight and relaxed, you can move on to some bicep hammer curls.

● Slowly raise your arms, either both together or one at a time—depending which you find easiest. Keep your elbows still and by your sides, as they are the points around which the movement pivots.

● Raise your arms as high as possible without moving your elbows. Then slowly lower them to the rest position by your sides. Use heavier weights to make the exercise more demanding but do not change your technique.

lunges with upper body *endurance*

Lunges require lots of balance and control. Be really careful when stepping, as it is easy to misjudge the exact distance of each step.

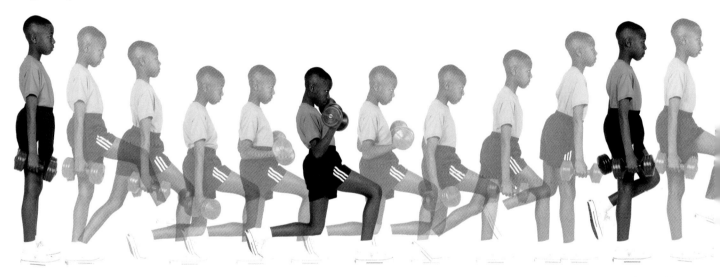

● Stand upright with a light weight in each hand. If the weight is too heavy, you will struggle to balance. If necessary, use no weight at all. Before you take your first step, look for a target on the floor to step toward.

● You should have a 90-degree angle at both legs in the base of each lunge as shown above. If you find this difficult, test out the correct distance before you begin. Now step to the target with your right leg.

● When your right foot touches the floor, stop moving and start to lower your body straight down. Stop when both knees are bent at 90 degrees. As you start this movement, begin the bicep curl with both arms.

● Return to the standing position and lower your arms to your sides. The next step forward is taken with the left leg. Again aim for a target and pause before lowering yourself into the lunge.

■   ▶   **breathe in**   ▶   **... out**

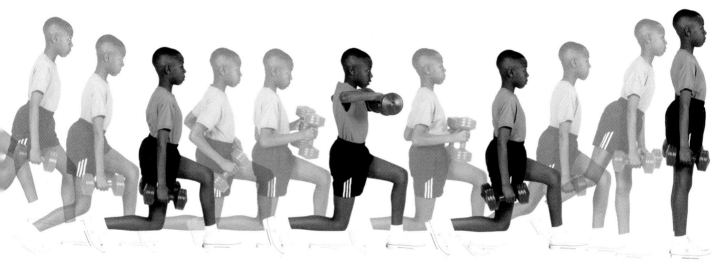

● This time, stop and hold the 90-degree position just a little way from the floor. Do this with a slow, controlled movement. Now bring your arms up into position for the shoulder exercise.

● Hold the lunge position and raise both arms out to the side; try to maintain a 90-degree angle with your elbows and knees. Lift both arms until they are level with your shoulders, as shown in the sequence above.

● Keep holding this difficult position. Then return both arms to your sides. Push up and step forward to the standing stance where you started. Always remember to repeat all the exercises evenly on both legs.

● If you want to make the exercise more difficult, you can either use heavier weights or complete more repetitions on each lunge. Remember to carry out the same number of repetitions on each leg.

▶ ... in   ▶ ... out   ... relax ■

dyna raise and squat *endurance*

Dyna bands come in different colors and strengths. There is no industry standard, and adult bands are much stronger than those intended for children.

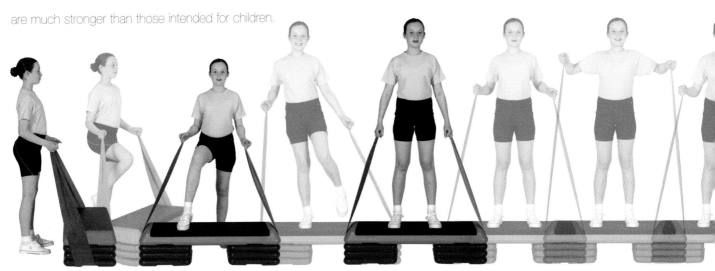

● The instructor must first check that the band is the appropriate strength and then set the step and bands correctly. Take hold of your bands in each hand and begin to lift your right leg onto the step.

● Now step up with the left leg, moving evenly onto the step with your feet wide apart. Before you start any exercise, check that the bands are taut and there is no slack.

● The first exercise is for the shoulders. Start to raise both your arms out to each side. You may be able to lift them evenly, or you may find that one is stronger than the other.

● Try to raise both your hands to shoulder height. If this is too difficult, bend both your arms at the elbows. This shortens your levers and makes it easier to raise your arms; the exercise is most difficult when they are straight.

■ ▶ **breathe in**   ▶   **... out**   ‖   **... in**   ▶   **... out**

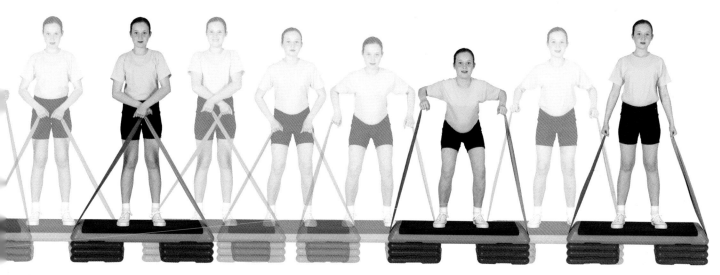

● Slowly return both arms to the starting position and cross them in front of the your lap. Once in this position, prepare for the second exercise, the squat. Combine this with the previous shoulder exercise.

● To do the squat, start by bending at both knees, pushing your lower body back and down as if you were sitting in a chair. Then lean your upper body forward to balance yourself but keep an upright posture.

● Lower yourself until you achieve a 90-degree angle at the knees. While squatting, raise your arms up to each side. Remember, if you bend your arms, the exercise is much easier than if you straighten them.

● Do not squat too deeply. Also, do not allow your body posture to slacken while repeating the exercise.

hamstring ball curl

This exercise is good for improving the hamstring muscles of the back of the thigh. The exercise requires a lot of balance and coordination if it is to be carried out correctly but can be varied so that it suitable for beginners and advanced users.

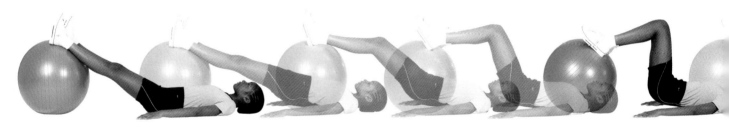

● Start by lying down on the floor on your ba.ck. Then place your feet on the ball about a hip's width apart in the center of the ball. Keep your legs straight with your feet pointing toward the ceiling.

● Move your hands out slightly from your body, as this helps you to balance. Now push your hips toward the ceiling, lifting your bottom, and lower back off the floor until your body is straight.

● Keep your feet pointing toward the ceiling and your hips raised. Then bend at both knees and roll the ball toward your bottom. If you find it difficult to balance, try taking your arms out wider.

● Keep rolling the ball toward you. Watch out for any changes in the position of your hips, keep your feet pointing toward the ceiling, and also try to keep your knees straight. Do not let them turn in or out.

■ ▶ **breathe in**   **... out**   ▶ **... out**

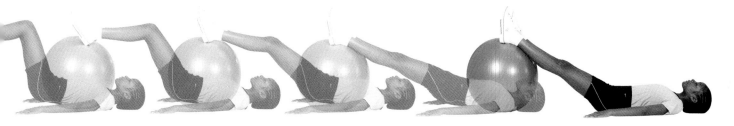

● When you are rolling the ball, try not to point your toes as if on tip toe; keep them relaxed. Roll the ball until your legs have reached a 90-degree angle at the knee. Then return the ball slowly to its starting position.

● When returning the ball, be careful to repeat the key points of the exercise. Continue to straighten your legs as you move to the start position, but do not drop your hips until you have finished all the repetitions.

● To rest, lower your bottom to the floor and relax. The exercise can be made harder if you move your feet together on the ball and put your hands close to your body, or even fold your arms over your chest.

● The hardest variation of the exercise is to cross one foot over the other. To make it easier, do not lift your bottom off the floor; just roll the ball back and forth with constant pressure.

... in   ▶   ... in   ▶   ... out, relax   ■

chest press and squat *endurance*

This simple exercise benefits both the upper and lower body and can be done anywhere. It helps to develop the muscles of the chest, shoulders, the back of the arms in the upper body, and the front and back muscles of the lower body.

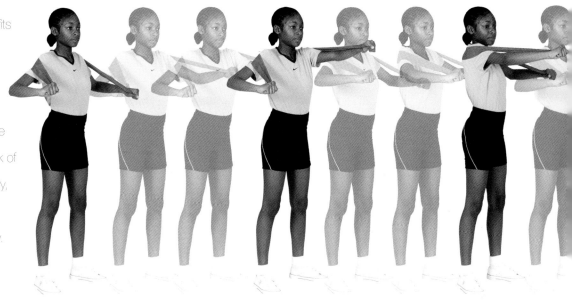

● Place the dyna band evenly across your upper back, roughly level with your shoulder blades. Your arms should be about mid-chest height: adjust the tension so there is no slack in the band.

● Stand up straight, keep your legs soft, and begin to push your left arm forward. Imagine that there is someone of the same height in front of you and try to touch his or her nose slowly.

● Return your left arm slowly to the starting position and do the same movement with your right. When using the arms separately like this, be careful not to twist your hips or over-reach and lean forward.

● Move your right arm back and prepare to stretch both arms together. At the same time, you are going to do a squat, so take your time to coordinate everything.

■　▶　**breathe in**　**… out**　▶　**… in, out**

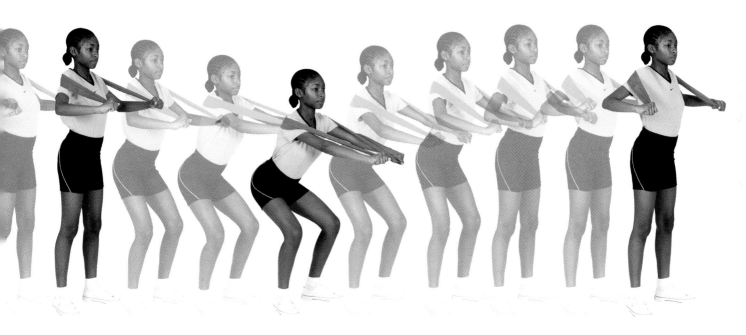

● Push both arms out in front of you. Even though you are squatting, imagine there is a person in front of you copying your squat, so you should still aim to touch their nose.

● Push your lower body back as if you were about to sit in a chair and, at the same time, lean forward with the upper part of your body to counterbalance your body weight.

● Lower yourself into the squat until your knees are bent at 90 degrees. Be careful not to allow your knees to go forward over your toes. Once you have reached the bottom of the squat, start to push up out of the position.

● As you stand up, return your arms to their resting position and resume the upright starting posture. Repeat the exercise as many times as you wish: to make it harder, use a stronger band.

▶　　　... in, out　　　　　　　　▶　　... out　　　　　　　▶　　　... in, out, relax　　　■

front raise and high row

These two exercises are designed for the upper body. The first, the front raise, works the shoulder muscles; the second, the high row, strengthens the muscles of the upper back and is an extremely good exercise for improving faulty posture.

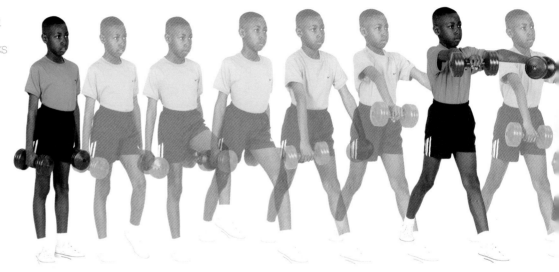

● Stand relaxed, with your hands by your sides. Tighten your stomach muscles ready for the first lift. Now step forward with your left leg, ready to brace your body.

● Lift both arms together directly in front of you. To make it easier, you can lift one at a time but remember not to twist your hips if you do this. Keep on lifting until your arms are level with your chin.

● If you are lifting weights in front of you with straight arms, you need to be careful with your back. If you feel any stress in your lower back, lighten the weight and tighten your abdominal muscles more.

■ ▶ **breathe in** ▶ **... out**

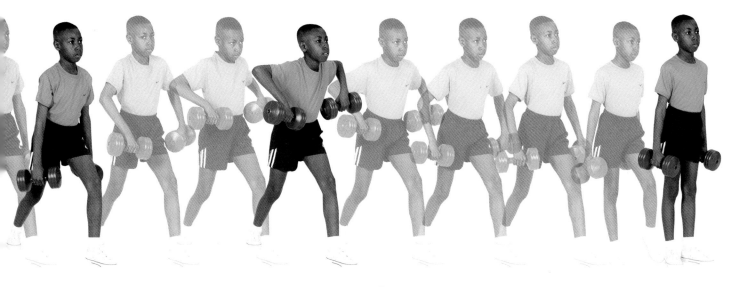

● Next, slowly lower the weights toward your knees. To progress to the second exercise, lean forward so your body is aligned with your back leg. There should be a straight line from your right heel to your head.

● Bring the dumbbells forward beside your knees. To start the exercise, squeeze your shoulder blades together and follow this by lifting your elbows up toward your shoulder blades.

● Keep lifting to a full squeeze and then slowly return the dumbbells to your knees. All the time you are doing this exercise, maintain that straight line between your right heel and your head.

● To finish, step forward and relax. If you want to try out these exercises, start by using a light weight. They are both very technical, so be careful: you could strain your back by doing them incorrectly.

▶ … in   ▶ … out   ▶ … relax

dyna press and extension

strength and endurance

This is another great exercise that can be done anywhere; it works the shoulder and back of the arm muscles. This exercise is quite difficult to coordinate because it uses both arms separately.

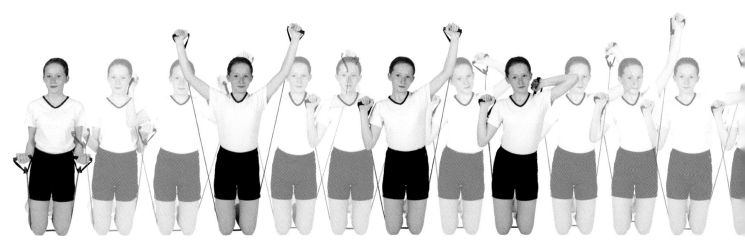

● Kneel down on a padded surface and remember to keep your body upright throughout the exercise. Trap the dyna band under your knees, hold it in each hand, and adjust the tension to suit your strength.

● The more firmly you trap the band, the harder the resistance will be and the sooner it will start. First, bring both arms up to shoulder height with your palms facing forward. Push both arms up toward the ceiling.

● Gently lower them to shoulder height. Then push up again, this time using only the left arm while the right rests. Keep pushing until your arm is almost straight.

● Pause in this position. Then lower your left arm, taking your hand down behind your head. Control this motion carefully and make sure your back remains straight.

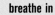 **breathe in** ▶  **... out** ▶  **... in** ▶ **... out**

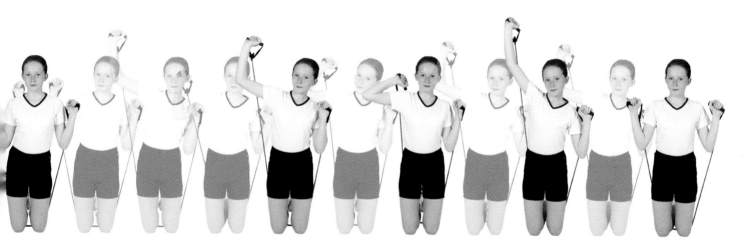

● Now push your left arm back up again toward the ceiling. When carrying out this movement, try to keep your right upper arm perfectly still. Only move your left arm.

● Check your posture and then repeat the exercise with your right arm. First, push it toward the ceiling, hold it still, then lower your arm behind your shoulder.

● Be careful not to twist your back or lean in any direction. Once your right arm is fully bent, as shown above, push it up as you did with your left arm. These two exercises can be done separately or together, as shown here.

● To finish, slowly lower your right arm down to the start position. To make the exercise harder, shorten the band. Be careful not to strain your back; concentrate on how your back is feeling during the exercise.

▶ ... in ▶ ... in ▶ ... out ▶ ... out, relax ■

arm dyna band pullover

This exercise works the muscles in the back of the arms, the upper sides of back, the chest, and shoulders. It requires a good range of flexibility in the shoulder area, so take it gently at first and only work to a range that feels comfortable. It is important not to overstrain your muscles when starting a new exercise.

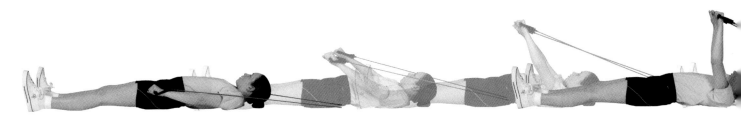

● Start by attaching the dyna band to an immovable object, such as a closed door. Then lie down on your back with the dyna band behind your head an arm's stretch away; there should be no slack in the dyna band.

● Pull the band down toward you on both sides of your body, with your palms facing toward the floor. Start the exercise slowly, controlling the action of raising your arms up and over your body.

● Keep your arms straight at all times. The exercise should look as if you are doing the backstroke, using both arms at the same time. Keep moving your arms back as they point toward the ceiling.

● Be careful doing this exercise if you have any shoulder problems. This is the point during the movement where there is a higher risk of injury to the joint. Keep moving back steadily against the resistance.

■ ▶ **breathe in** ▶ ▶ … in

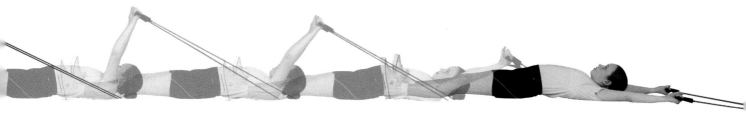

● As your arms go back and get closer to the floor, the resistance decreases. If the exercise seems too easy, position yourself slightly farther away from the band to increase the stretch.

● It is possible to do this exercise using one arm at a time. If you try this, make sure that your lower back doesn't twist or lift off the floor, which it will have a tendency to do.

● If your back does twist or lift, stop before you touch the floor and take the band back above your head with straight arms.

● Once you have completed the desired number of repetitions, lower your arms to the floor above your head and rest.

▶   **... out**   ▶   ▶   **... out, relax**   ■

ball abdominal crunch

This is the first abdominal exercise. It works the front abdominal muscles from the sternum to the pelvis. This exercise is very versatile and suitable for both beginner and advanced students. To make it easier, sit further forward over the ball: to make it harder, sit further back.

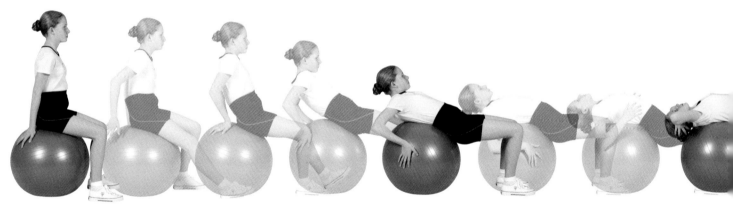

● Start by sitting on the ball with your weight in the center. Place your feet a hip's width apart and your hands the same distance apart on the back of the ball. This helps you to balance properly.

● Starting with your left leg, begin to move forward slowly and, at the same time, lean back, transferring more of your weight on to your arms. Then, do the same with your right leg.

● Lean further back onto your hands to support your body weight and continue your forward movement until you feel the lumber lower arch of your back touch the ball.

● At this point, you should be lying on the top of the ball. Take your hands away from the ball and bring them up to your head to support your neck.

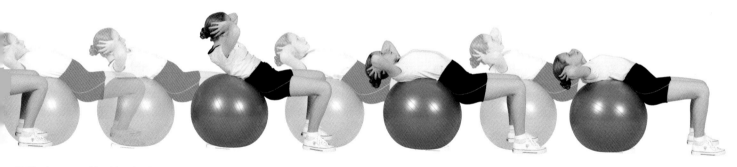

● Check your position. You should be completely relaxed with most of your body weight on your lower back, your feet a hip's width apart, and your knees bent at 90 degrees.

● To make the exercise harder, push back further over the ball. To begin the crunch, lift your head and shoulders, using your abdominal muscles only. Do not pull your head up with your hands; this might strain your neck muscles.

● When carrying out the crunch, keep your body weight centered on your lower back. To do this, you may have to lift your hips up to the ceiling so that your body stays straight.

● When you have crunched as far as possible, slowly lower yourself back until you are right over the ball. After several repetitions, use your hands to help you sit upright.

▶ ... out   ... out   ▶ ... in   ▶ ... out, relax

dorsal raise

This is an excellent work out for the muscles in the lower part of the back. It can be quite a gentle exercise but can be done in two ways to give different levels of intensity; you can either do it on your knees (not illustrated) or, the harder version, on your feet.

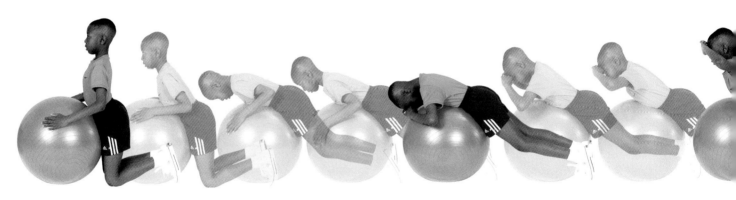

● Start by kneeling down on a padded floor with the ball directly in front of you and your body upright. Keep your knees and feet a hip's width apart at all times.

● Now lean forward, placing your stomach on the ball; use your hands to keep the ball still. Then start to push from your feet and begin to lift your knees off the floor.

● Keep pushing from your feet until your legs are almost straight—your position is very important. The further forward you are and the more weight you have on your hips, the harder the exercise becomes.

● Now bring your hands in front of you and position them so that you can rest your head on them. Before you start the main part of the exercise, relax over the ball and check that your feet are apart.

■ ▶ **breathe in**　　　▶ **... in**　　　▶ **... out**

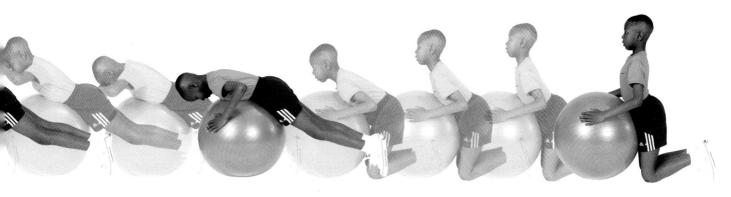

● Lift yourself up as high as possible, using your lower back muscles. Always do this exercise as slowly and smoothly as you can to minimize the chance of injury.

● When you have reached as high as you can, pause for a second to help you control the lowering phase of the exercise. During the whole exercise, try not to use any other muscles than those in your lower back.

● After a few repetitions, bring your hands down onto the ball and drop your knees slowly toward the floor. When your knees touch the floor, push yourself upright into the starting position with your hands.

● Be careful not to move too far forward on the ball, as you are likely to roll over the front.

▶ ... out   ▶ ... in   ▶ ... out, relax   ■

dyna band twist

strength and endurance

This is an advanced exercise to increase core stability—the strength and balance of the torso

muscles. It works the entire abdomen and all back muscles and is very good for improving posture.

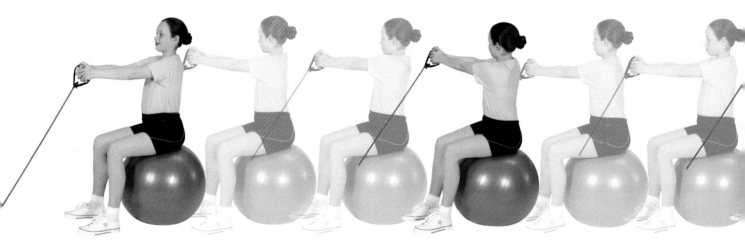

● Start by attaching the dyna band to an immovable object. Then sit on the ball far enough away that there is no slack in the band. Sit in the center of the ball with your feet a hip's width apart.

● The band should be directly in front of you with your arms at shoulder height and your head level, facing the front. Now begin to turn from the waist only, not from the arms or hips.

● Look for a target point and then start to turn to the right. When turning, keep your body upright and keep your abdominal muscles pulled in tight.

● Keep turning as far as possible, remembering to turn from the waist only, and without moving the ball. Once you have fully rotated, with your arms still straight out in front of you, gently return to the starting position.

■ **breathe in**    **... out**

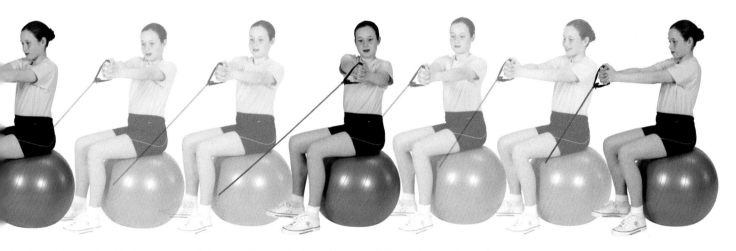

● Repeat the exercise, this time turning to the left. If you want to increase the intensity of the exercise, either sit further away from the anchor point of the band or bring your feet closer together.

● Once you have reached your full rotation again, slowly return toward the center. When doing this exercise, remember to keep your arms out in front of your chest all the time and only turn from your waist.

● Repeat the exercise as often as you wish but pause in the center before each turn to check your position and posture.

● Once you have done enough, relax and slowly let go of the dyna band. For a more advanced work-out, lift one foot off the floor when turning. Remember to change feet on each side.

▶ **pause, breathe in, out** ▶ **... out** ▶ **... in** ▶ **... out, relax**

core stability exercise *endurance*

This exercise is a little easier than the one shown on pages 64–65. Here, there is more emphasis on the back muscles than on the stomach. Although the exercise is easier, it does require more balance and has two levels of difficulty. The easier version is the one featured, although the harder version is also explained in the text.

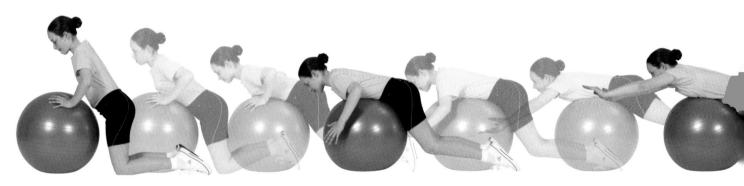

● Kneel down on a padded floor with your hands on the ball to help you balance while you get into the correct starting position.

● Slowly lean forward so that your stomach is on the ball. Slide your hands down either side. All your weight should be supported by the ball and your feet should be a hip's width apart.

● Start to push forward with both legs. You are aiming to push yourself forward over the top of the ball until you are balanced. Be careful not to roll over the front.

● When you are in this position, your legs should be straight. Now take both your hands off the ball and hold them straight out in front of your head as shown above.

■   **breathe in**   ▶   … **in**   ▶   … **out**

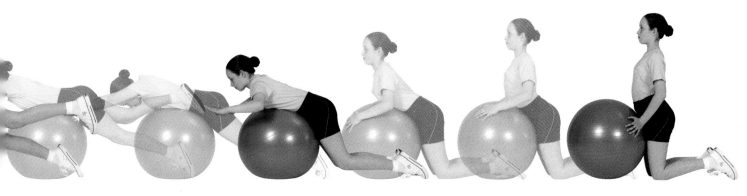

● At the same time, raise your left leg about 12in (30cm) from the floor and hold this position for about 30 seconds. Then change legs, lifting the right one. Again, hold this position for 30 seconds.

● If you want to try a harder version of this exercise, lift both legs off the floor at the same time and hold for 30 seconds. Repeat the exercise as many times as you wish.

● When you have finished, gently come out of the exercise. Slowly lower your knees down to the floor and bring your hands back onto the ball to help you push yourself upright.

● Lean away from the ball and kneel upright. During the exercise, keep your abdominal muscles tight and breathe constantly to help you relax and control your balance when you are on the ball.

▶   ... out   ▶   ... in   ▶   ... out, relax   ■

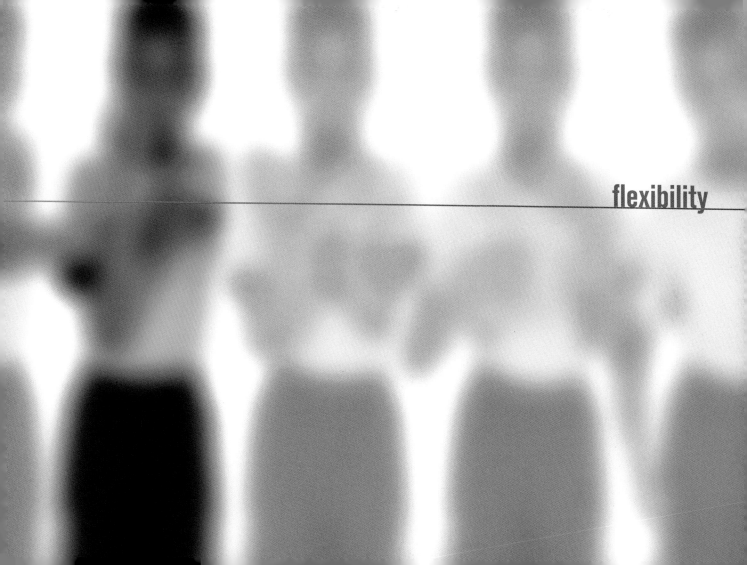

flexibility

calf, back, and chest

flexibility

This spread demonstrates three different stretches that are usually done as a warm-up before any resistance or aerobic workout. The stretches are quick and easy to do, as they are combined with each other. If you find that you have trouble doing them together, they can be done individually. Start with one and then add the other two as you become more flexible.

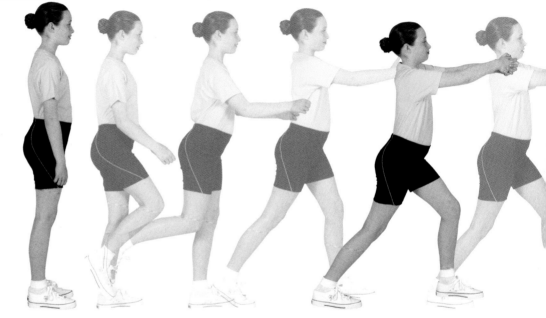

● Stand in a relaxed position with your arms by your side. Lift your right leg off the floor and step back, keeping the weight on your left leg. At the same time, start to lift both your arms out in front of you.

● Make sure that the step with your right leg is a long one and a bit of a reach, as your toes must touch the ground first. At this point, your arms should be at chest height with your hands together.

● Now push your right heel to the floor to feel the stretch in your right calf. If you do not feel the stretch, then shuffle your right foot further back until you can feel it. Make sure your foot is always facing forward.

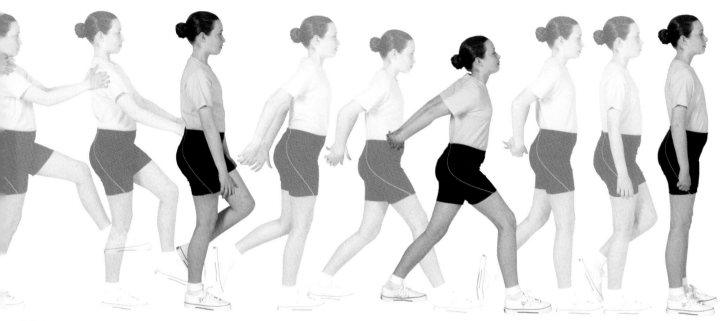

● Push your arms forward as far as possible but maintain an upright posture. You should feel a stretch in your upper back. Hold both stretches for at least 20 seconds and then release your arms and start to step back.

● Step back with your left leg, planting it well back behind your right. Make sure it is a bit of a reach before you plant your foot. Move your arms behind you, ready to grasp your hands behind your back.

● Plant your left heel on the floor and feel the stretch. If not, shuffle back a bit further as before. Grasp you hands together, straighten both arms, and lift them up behind you.

● Keep your body upright. You will now feel the stretch across your shoulders and chest. Hold both positions for 20 seconds, then relax. Step forward and bring your legs together, arms relaxed by your sides.

gluteals cross legs

Here we have two stretches for the gluteals, the muscles of the bottom. It is very important to keep the gluteals flexible, as they are powerful muscles with a strong influence on posture and stress in the whole lower back region. Keeping the gluteals flexible is a means of minimizing stress and tightness around the lower back, and reduces the chance of future posture problems.

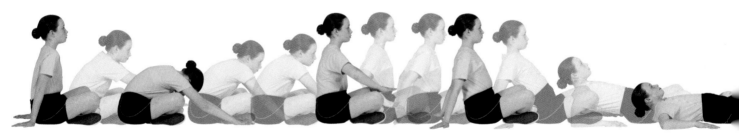

● Start by sitting with your legs crossed and your feet under your knees. Place your hands behind you to help keep your posture upright. You may already feel a stretch and, if so, stay in this position for 20 seconds.

● The stretch should come on either side of your bottom. If you cannot feel it, lean further forward and hold. Note that very flexible people may not feel the stretch even when they are leaning fully forward.

● Check that you feel the stretch on both sides. If not, you may need to swap your crossed legs over. Then repeat the exercise. Pause and relax. Then lie down on your back, using your hands for support.

● Now uncross your legs, placing your left ankle on your right knee with your right leg bent at 90 degrees and your foot flat on the floor.

 ▶ **breathe in**   ‖ ▶ **... out**   ▶ **... in and out**   **... in and out**

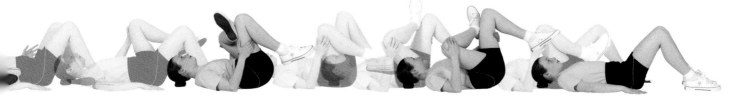

● Put your right hand around your right thigh and your left hand on your left knee. Slowly pull your right knee toward your chest until you feel a stretch in your left buttock.

● Hold the stretch for 20 seconds, then release. Swap your legs and hands over so that your right ankle is on your left knee. Repeat the stretch.

● This time, pull your left knee in as far as possible and you will feel the stretch in your right buttock. Hold this for about 20 seconds. Now release the stretch, let go with your hands, and put them on the floor beside you.

● Put your feet flat on the floor with your legs bent at 90 degrees. If you have trouble performing the first stretch in this sequence, sit up against a wall and use your hands to push yourself into a deep stretch.

  ... in and out ❚❚ ▶  **... in** ❚❚ **... out** ▶ **... in and out, relax** ■

quadriceps

This exercise stretches the
quadriceps muscles that run
down the front of your thigh.
The stretch itself is quite
simple, but if you have any
sort of knee problem, it must
be approached with care.
It is easy to compress the
knee joint if this stretch is
done incorrectly and this
can aggravate any
existing injuries.

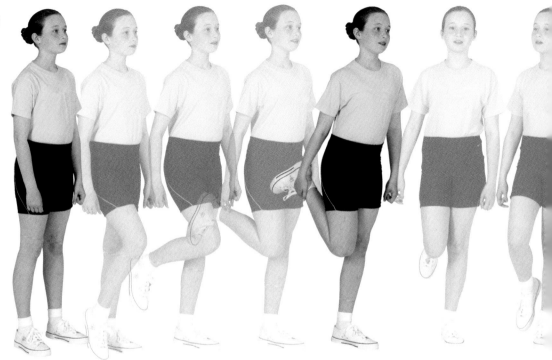

● Stand upright with your arms by
your sides. Then begin to lift your right
foot up behind you toward your
bottom. While doing this, prepare
to grab hold of your leg at the ankle
with your right hand as shown.

● When you have a firm hold of
your ankle, pull your foot up behind
you. Do not press it against your
bottom, as this will over-compress
your knee joint.

● Keep your knees together.
You should feel the stretch down the
front of your thigh. To increase it, push
your hips forward away from your
foot, increasing the gap between it and
your bottom.

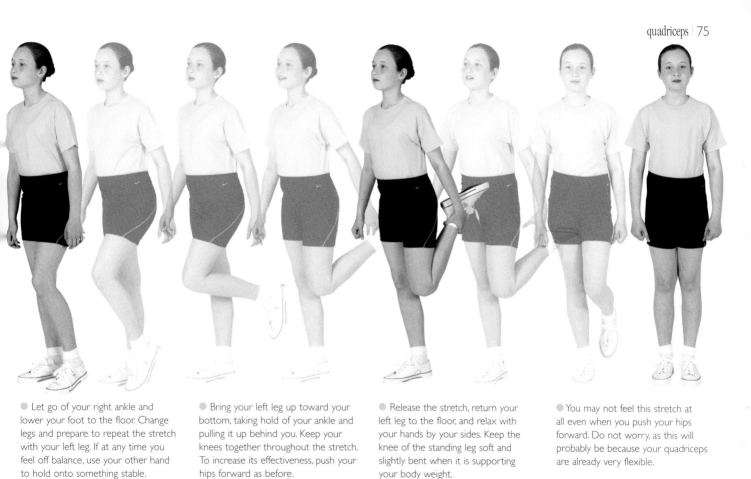

● Let go of your right ankle and lower your foot to the floor. Change legs and prepare to repeat the stretch with your left leg. If at any time you feel off balance, use your other hand to hold onto something stable.

● Bring your left leg up toward your bottom, taking hold of your ankle and pulling it up behind you. Keep your knees together throughout the stretch. To increase its effectiveness, push your hips forward as before.

● Release the stretch, return your left leg to the floor, and relax with your hands by your sides. Keep the knee of the standing leg soft and slightly bent when it is supporting your body weight.

● You may not feel this stretch at all even when you push your hips forward. Do not worry, as this will probably be because your quadriceps are already very flexible.

▶ … in   ❚❚ ▶ … out   ▶ … in and out, relax ■

hamstrings

This is a relaxation stretch; done lying on your back, your heart rate will remain low. The hamstrings need stretching regularly to maintain their length, as they are one of the major postural muscles of the lower back and pelvis. The stretch is shown here using a dyna band (you could use a towel) to make it easier for you to reach your leg, but if you are quite flexible, then you should be able to reach without it.

● Start by lying on your back with the dyna band attached to the heel of your left foot and both your arms and legs straight. You should be holding each end of the dyna band in your hands.

● Slowly lift your left leg, bending your knee toward your chest. Make sure the dyna band tracks this movement, pulling on the band as your leg comes up.

● When your leg reaches about 90 degrees at your hip, raise your foot into the air, using your quadriceps muscles and pulling on the dyna band. Straighten it as much as you can, depending on your flexibility.

● The aim is to straighten your leg completely at 90 degrees to the ground without your resting leg lifting off the floor. You should feel the stretch in the middle of your hamstring and not behind your knee.

■ ▶ **breathe in** ▶ **... out** ❚❚

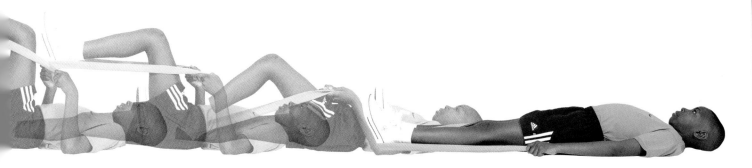

● If you do feel the stretch behind your knee, bend your leg slightly. This helps to transfer the stretch to your hamstring. Once you feel the desired stretch, hold the position for 20 seconds.

● Release your left leg, lowering it to the floor. Repeat the stretch on your right leg in the same way, bringing your knee up until it is at 90 degrees to your hip first. Then straighten your leg until you feel the stretch.

● Only straighten your leg enough to feel the stretch in the middle of your thigh. If you start to feel the stretch behind your knee, bend your leg slightly as before.

● When in the stretch position, avoid lifting the other leg off the floor. If this happens, you are pulling your leg too far toward your chest. Finally, keep your feet relaxed at all times and do not point or flex your toes.

▶ ...in

▶ ... in, out

▶ ... out, relax

hips and triceps

The main stretch is to the hip flexor muscles in the front at the top of the thigh. The other stretch is of the triceps at the back of the arm.

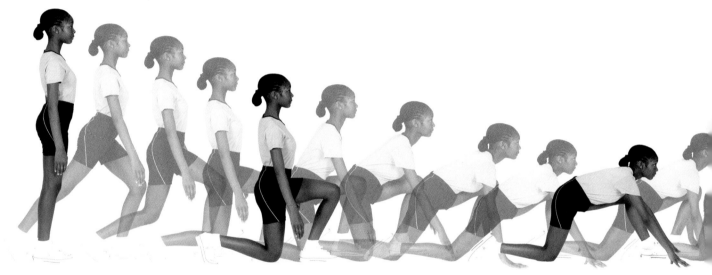

● Start by standing upright. Then step back and reach with your right leg. Lower your right knee toward the floor to the kneeling position, bending your left leg.

● You should now be kneeling on your right knee with both legs bent at approximately 90 degrees. Keep your body upright. You may start to feel the stretch at the top of the front of your right thigh.

● To increase the stretch, lean forward and place your hands on the floor to balance yourself. Then slide your left leg forward, increasing the angle between your legs.

● The further you move your left leg forward, the more you will feel the stretch. Hold and then sit upright, putting your hands on your left knee.

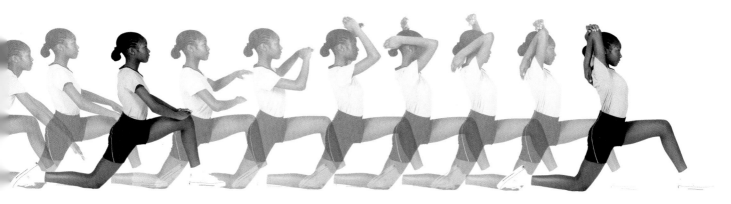

● To further increase the stretch, lean further forward and slide your left foot forward again. When stretching your hip flexors, always try to keep both hips facing forward; do not let them turn to the right.

● The second phase stretches the triceps. Take your right arm up behind your head and reach down toward the center of your back. Bring your left arm up and over your head, taking hold of your right elbow.

● Start to pull your right arm further down the center of your back. You should feel the stretch in the middle of the back of your right arm.

● Hold both positions for 20 seconds. To increase the hip flexor stretch, tilt your pelvis forward and tighten your abdominal muscles. When stretching the triceps, try not to lean too far back. Repeat on the other leg and arm.

… in    … out   … in    …out    relax

inner thighs

This exercise stretches the muscles in the inner thighs. Depending on your flexibility, it can also stretch the muscles either side of the lower back and the hamstrings. The stretch has three aims: first, to open the legs wider; second, to lean further forward; and third, to lean further to each side. This sequence shows the three key positions and should be done in the order demonstrated.

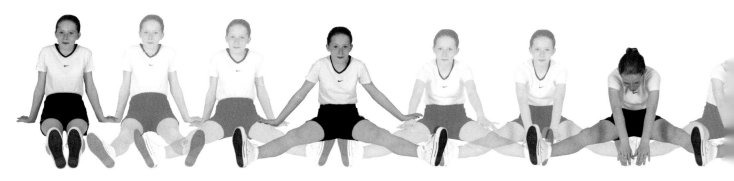

● Sit with your legs out in front, feet together, with your hands on either side of your body for support. Push yourself into an upright position.

● Move your legs apart, as wide as possible. You should feel an even stretch running down the inside of both thighs. The stretch should be felt most by your knees.

● Relax into this stretch and then progress to the next position. Bring both your hands forward onto the floor between your thighs. Relax, take deep breaths, and slowly lean forward.

● Every time you feel the stretch ease, lean further forward. As you do this, the stretch will move higher up your inner thighs toward the groin area. Once you cannot go any further, move on to the next stretch.

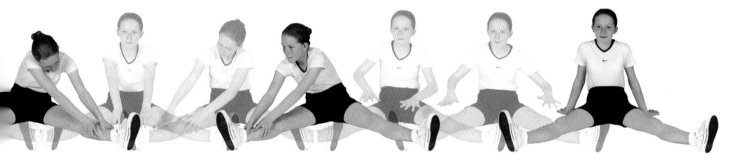

● With your hands together, slide them down your left leg to your left ankle. This will increase the stretch on your left inner thigh and may create a stretch on the left side of your lower back and left hamstring.

● Once you can hold your ankle with both hands, lean forward, bringing your chest down over your left thigh. Once you have pushed as far as you can on the left, repeat this stretch on your right side.

● Push the stretch on the right as far as you can go, bringing your chest down over your right thigh. Hold this position for 20 seconds.

● Relax, put both arms behind you, and sit upright, facing forward. Put both your hands on the floor and use them as support to help you sit up properly.

❙❙   ▶   ... in and out   ▶   ... in and out   ❙❙   ▶   ... in and out, relax   ■

back lateral stretch

flexibility

This exercise stretches the upper back and torso muscles. It also mobilizes the lower vertebrae, lubricating each of the major joints.

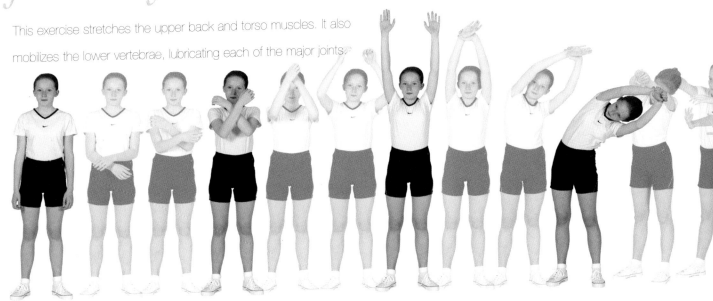

● Stand upright with your arms by your sides. Bring your arms in front of your body, crossing them over at your waist. Then take them up together toward your face.

● Keep pushing your arms up, opening them out above your head by pushing them up toward the ceiling. Reach straight above you for the first stretch.

● Push as hard as possible toward the ceiling and feel your upper body elongating. Take hold of your right wrist with your left hand, and staying stretched out, lean to your left side.

● Lean over as far as possible and only lean to the left, not forward or back. Pull your right arm with your left hand to increase the stretch down your right side and waist.

■ ▶ **breathe in**   **… in**   ❚❚ ▶ **… out**   ❚❚ ▶ **… in and out**

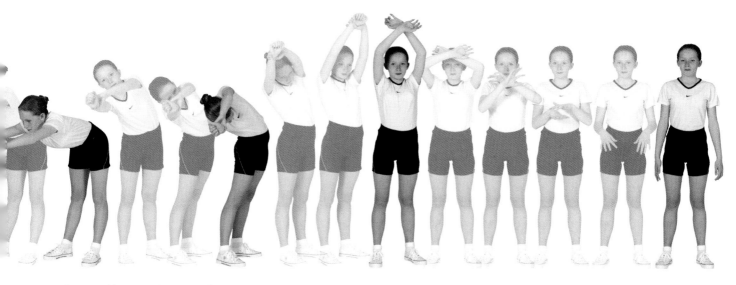

● Keep pulling yourself over and then start to lean forward, rolling from your hips. Keep your body at the same angle as you move. Release your right arm and push your bottom back to feel a stretch in your hamstrings.

● Roll across to your right side, transferring the stretch from your hamstrings to the left side of your waist and upper back. Use your right hand to pull your left arm over to increase the stretch as shown.

● Stand upright, release your left arm, and push up toward the ceiling in the same way that you started the exercise. You can now repeat the stretch, rolling in the opposite direction.

● Finally, bring your hands down, crossing them in front of your face and uncrossing them at the waist as shown. Return to the relaxed starting position.

❚❚ ▶ ... in and out   ... in and out ❚❚   ▶ ... in   ▶ ... out, relax ◼

ball back extension

This exercise requires the use of a ball and should be done with caution if you have any sort of back problem. Be very gentle when you start doing this exercise; although with practice, it will improve the flexibility and health of your spine.

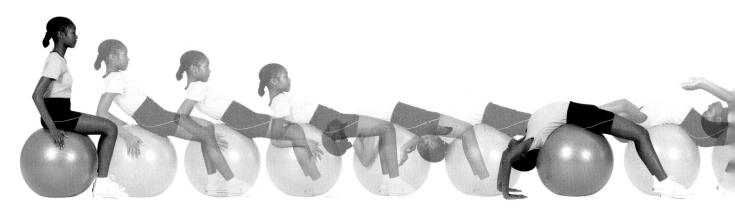

● Sit on the ball with your hands on either side of your body to help you keep your balance. You should be sitting upright with your knees bent at 90 degrees, your feet wide apart and flat on the floor.

● Walk your feet forward, starting with your right foot. As you do this, lean on your hands, sliding your body down onto the ball. Keep walking forward until the small of your lower back touches the surface of the ball.

● Let your arms slide down the ball; your body should now be resting on the ball. Put your head back and relax. You may already feel a stretch in your abdominal muscles.

● If the stretch is too hard, walk your feet forward. If the stretch is too weak, slide your hands around behind your head and push back further, straightening your legs, and supporting your bottom with the ball.

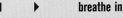 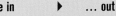 breathe in … out  … in  … out

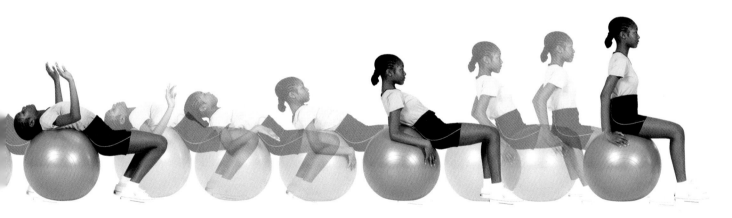

● You will also feel a release of any stiffness in your lower back. Slowly roll the ball forward and bring your arms up and over, transferring all your weight to your legs. Put your hands back on the ball as shown.

● Pause for a second or two to allow the blood to flow down away from your head; then push yourself upright. Roll the ball back to help you return to the sitting position.

● Return to the sitting position, just as you started, and relax. Note that when doing this exercise, all movements should be slow and smooth. When you are in the stretch position, use your hands to balance.

● Keep your feet wide apart at all times. If you have been lying in this position for a while, you may feel stiffness in your lower back when sitting up. If so, follow this exercise with the one on pages 86–87.

▶   ... in   ▶   ... out, pause, in   ▶   ... out, relax

rotational flexibility

This exercise stretches the muscles of the torso, which are often stiff because of inactivity. It also mobilizes and lubricates the spine and is also very good for removing or reducing tension in the lower back.

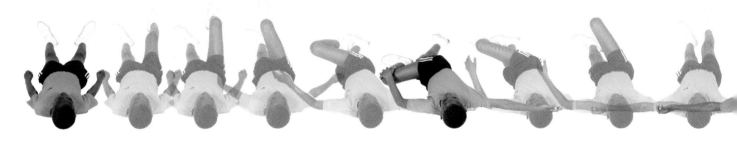

● To start this exercise, lie down flat on your back with your arms by your sides. First, lift your right leg up toward your chest until it reaches an angle of 90 degrees at your right hip.

● Keeping your leg at 90 degrees at the hip, roll your right knee over the left side of your body toward the floor. As you do this, slide your arms out to each side until they are just below your shoulders.

● Put your left hand on your right knee and pull your knee toward the floor; the aim while pressing is to keep your right shoulder flat on the floor. Press until you feel a good stretch or your right shoulder starts to lift.

● Feel the stretch across your torso, back, and side of your bottom. The optimum level for this exercise would be to have both your right knee and shoulder on the floor without feeling stretched.

■ ▶ **breathe in**　　　　　　▶　　　　　　Ⅱ　▶　… in　　　▶　… in

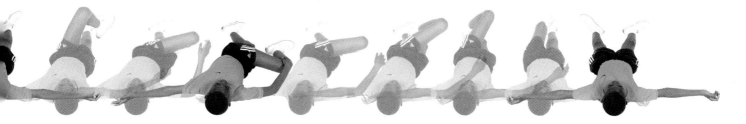

● Slowly, release your right knee and gently roll out of the stretch to the center and put your right leg down flat on the floor. At the same time, lift your left leg up to an angle of 90 degrees at the hip.

● Roll your left knee over your right leg and place your right hand on your left knee, ready to pull down. Slide your left arm out for balance and pull down into a good stretch.

● Hold the stretch for about 20 seconds on both sides; then roll your left hip back again, straightening your left leg down toward the floor. Allow your hips to relax and settle with your body flat on the floor.

● If you are feeling at all stiff, bring both knees up toward your chest and roll them together gently from left to right repeatedly until the stiffness is gone. This movement is not demonstrated above.

▶   ... in   ❚❚ ▶   ... out   ▶   ... in and out, relax   ■

shoulder and neck stretch

These stretches release tension in the upper back and neck. They are usually used for relaxation before and after exercise.

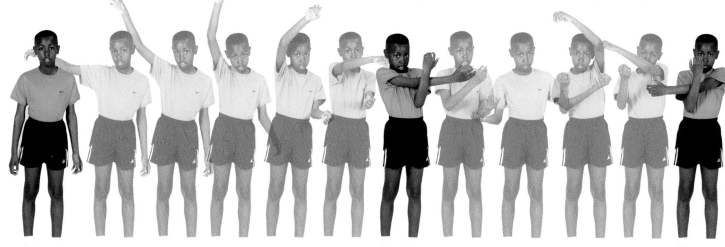

● Stand upright with your feet apart and your hands down by your sides. Start by lifting your right arm up and out to your right and keep going until it comes up and over, then down in front of your face.

● As your right arm comes down to shoulder level, take your left arm and bring it up in front of your right arm, so the inside of your left arm meets your right arm just above the elbow.

● Trap your right arm with your left and squeeze it into you. You will feel a stretch in the back of your right shoulder. Now release both arms and bring them down to your sides.

● Take your left arm up over your head and then down in front of your face until it is level with your shoulders. Bring your right arm up in front of your left and repeat the trap and squeeze.

■ ▶ **breathe in**   ▶ **... out and in**   ‖ ▶ **... out**   ▶ **... in and out**

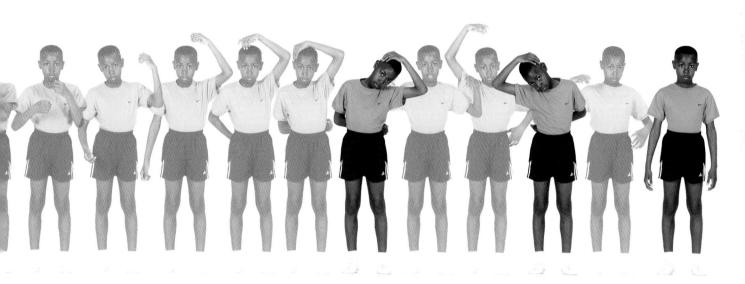

● Feel the stretch in the back of the left shoulder. Now let both arms drop to your waist and get ready to move on to the neck stretches. Lower your right arm to your side and bring your left one up and over your head.

● Take hold of the right side of your head with your left hand, as shown. At the same time, take your right arm and put it behind your back and hook it onto the left side of your waist.

● Pull your head gently to the left with your left arm and feel the stretch on the right side of your neck. Hold the stretch, then release. Change hands and then repeat the stretch on the other side.

● This time pull your head gently to the right with your right arm. Feel the stretch in the left side of your neck while the left arm is hooked into the right side of your waist. Then lower your arms to your sides and relax.

▶ ... in, relax   ▶ ... in   ‖ ▶ ... out   ... in and out ‖ ▶ ... in, out and relax ■

flexibility upper body mobilization

This exercise loosens, relaxes, and stretches most of the muscles in the upper body, including the neck, back, chest, and shoulders. It also warms those muscles and lubricates the shoulders, elbows, and spine. It is excellent for warming up before undertaking any strenuous routine.

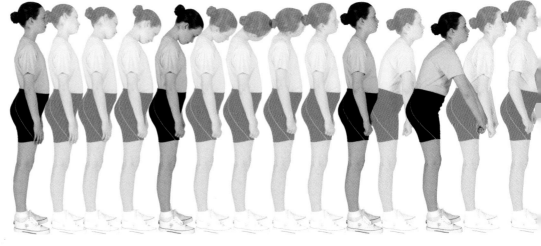

● Stand with your arms by your side and start by rolling your head to your left and then around toward the front. As you roll, dip your head toward your chest and face down to the floor.

● Continue the roll over to your right side and then back to the starting position. Repeat this exercise if necessary. These small rotations stretch and mobilize the neck area.

● Next, lean forward slightly and bring your hands together in front of you. Round your shoulders forward as shown and push your upper back outward. You will feel the stretch in your upper back area.

■   ▶ **breathe in**   ▶ **... out**   ▶ **... in and out   ... in**

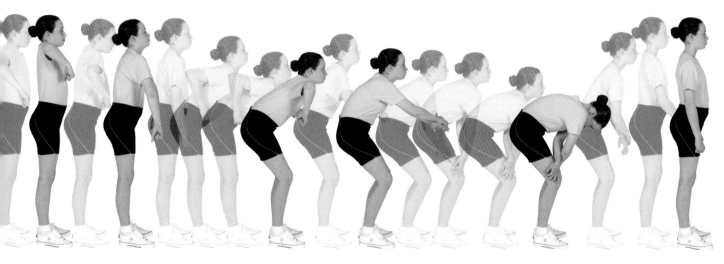

● From here, stand upright and pull your shoulders and arms back to open up your chest. You will feel the stretch across your chest and shoulders. Now stand up and lift your arms and elbows up toward your ears.

● Hold your arms in this position, lean forward, and then roll your elbows and shoulders over to round your upper back. This mobilizes the shoulders and stretches the upper back area.

● Next, push your hands out in front of you and straighten your arms to increase the stretch in your upper back area. Cross your arms and bend down slightly, placing each hand on the opposite leg.

● Pull against your legs. This increases the stretch in your upper back. Release your arms and stand up straight with your arms by your sides.

▶ ... out

▶ ... in, out

▶ ... in, out

▶ ... in, out, relax ■

lower body mobilization

This exercise stretches most of the lower back muscles and also those surrounding the hip area. At the same time, it mobilizes the lower back and hip joints, improving their health and range of movement. If you want, you can repeat the last two movements of the exercise a number of times until you feel completely loose and supple.

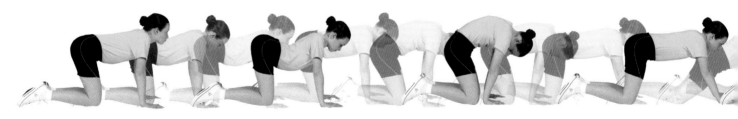

- Start by kneeling on all fours with your hands directly below your shoulders and your knees directly below your hips. Allow you lower back to "sit" in a neutral posture.

- Start to mobilize the lower back by pushing your stomach to the floor and making a concave arch with your back, as shown. Push as hard as you comfortably can before returning to the neutral position.

- Push your upper back up to the ceiling and slide your hands in toward your knees. This increases the mobility in your lower back, starts mobilizing your upper back, and stretches the upper back muscles.

- Hold this stretch, then slide your hands forward, supporting your body while lowering your hips toward the floor. Keep your arms straight at all times while you push your hips to the floor.

■ ▶ **breathe in**　　▶ **... out**　　▶ **... in**　　▶ **... out**

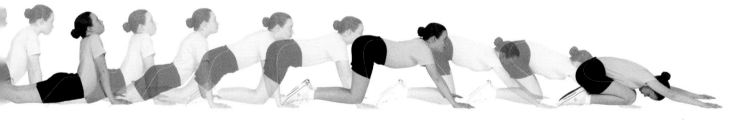

● Press your hips into the floor and push your lower back into an arch as shown above. Look up to the ceiling. You should feel your lower back relaxing as you hold this position.

● Lift your hips and push your bottom up and back over your knees. Slide your hands back as you do this. Keep sliding back until your bottom is sitting on your calves.

● Your head and arms should be stretched out in front of you as shown above. This mobilizes your lower back and reduces or removes any tension in the lower back area. Stay in this position until you feel relaxed.

● If you still feel any tension, repeat the last two movements, back and forth, until you are fully mobilized and relaxed (this is not shown above). You can also repeat the entire sequence if you wish.

▶   ... in, out   ▶   ... in   ▶   ▶   ... out, relax   ■

index

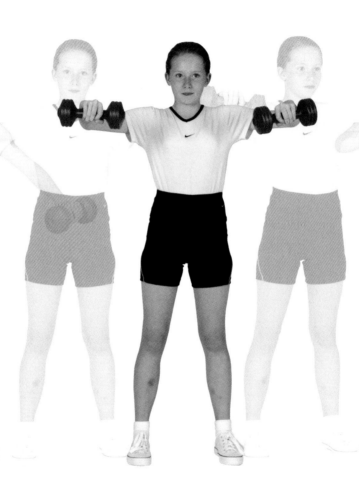

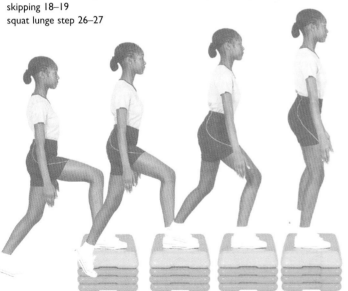

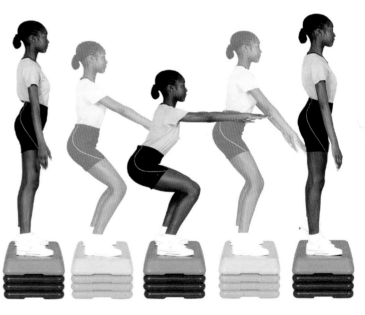